On the Cause and Treatment of Chronic Fatigue Syndrome

One Patient's Journey with His Doctor

by Robert Roy

Medical Disclaimer: As the author of this book, I freely state that I am not a licensed medical professional, and that the information shared here is based on personal experience. So the content of this book is for informational purposes only; it is not meant to provide or replace professional medical advice; and it is not intended to be used to diagnose, treat, cure, or prevent any condition or disease independent of professional medical oversight. This means you understand that this book is not intended as a substitute for consultation with a licensed medical practitioner. Please consult with your own physician or healthcare specialist regarding the information, suggestions and recommendations made in this book. The use of this book implies your acceptance of this disclaimer.

Table Of Contents

"Breakthroughs happen when limiting thoughts and behaviors are challenged."

— Fabienne Fredrickson: business mentor, writer/speaker.

Introduction

A dozen years before 2024, an amazing thing happened in regard to the illness of Chronic Fatigue Syndrome (CFS). My CFS specialist — Dr. Joseph Brewer of Kansas City, Missouri — theorized that toxic mold played a significant role in CFS. Then, by means of a newly available test, he preceded to find that toxic mold was present in a vast majority of his CFS patients. This result was soon duplicated by two other CFS specialists, on opposite coasts in the U.S., in their own medical practices. (The other two doctors were Dr. Paul Cheney in Asheville, North Carolina, and Dr. Neil Nathan in Northern California.)

So circa 2012, these three doctors tested their patients for toxic mold infection; and the test they used was very accurate, and one that never gave a false positive. And over a two year period, approximately 90% of the patients in each of these three doctor's medical practices tested positive for toxic mold.

Finally, in Dr. Brewer's medical practice, he proceeded to treat those patients of his who had tested positive for toxic mold with standard antifungal medications. From that treatment, and depending on which drug was used, approximately 83% to 94%

of those patients treated showed significant improvement or got completely well.

This book, then, is about (a) this startling discovery of the role toxic mold plays in CFS that was made by Dr. Brewer; (b) the discovery of another syndrome, Mast Cell Activation Syndrome (MCAS), that can also play a major role in CFS; (c) the treatments that Dr. Brewer has developed, or that are available, to treat these and other aspects of CFS; and (d) the success of these treatments.

Who is Dr. Brewer?

Dr. Joseph Brewer is board certified in internal medicine, and he has a private medical practice in Kansas City, Missouri. When the author began seeing the doctor regularly, according to the author's research from around that time, Dr. Brewer was also (a) the Medical Director of Infection Control and Hospital Epidemiology at Saint Luke's Hospital (which is a private teaching institution that is also involved in scientific and medical research), and (b) a Clinical Assistant Professor of Medicine at the University of Missouri at Kansas City School of Medicine.

The Information in this Book:

Most of this book is filled with the words spoken by Dr. Brewer during regular medical appointments with the author. These visits, beginning in 2011, usually were of a one hour duration and occurred twice a year.

As to the quotes attributed to Dr. Brewer, they are, in fact, not quite exact quotes. They've been edited by the author in order to move Dr. Brewer's spoken words into print, and they've also been edited for clarity.

Also, when Dr. Brewer mentions his CFS patients in this book, he is certainly referring to his fibromyalgia and chronic Lyme disease patients as well. In addition, Dr. Brewer doesn't distinguish CFS from Myalgic Encephalomyelitis (ME).

Furthermore, the author has edited his own notes that he presented to the doctor at the beginning of each office visit for both relevance and clarity.

Finally, in conversations in the book, the author is indicated by the names of either *Robert* or *Bob*.

<u>The Author:</u>

At the beginning of these office visits in 2012, I was a 67 year old white male. I'd had a career in accounting and finance until I had become too sick to work in early 1995.

I originally became chronically ill in October 1993, and in the following year I was diagnosed by Dr. Brewer with CFS. However, I didn't see Dr. Brewer again until I became a regular patient of the doctor's in 2005.

Robert Roy

As for Dr. Brewer, he has been practicing medicine since 1976. So in 2012, it appeared he was about 61 years old.

My Health Situation in Mid-2011:

a. I had all the major symptoms associated with CFS: extreme fatigue, post-exertional malaise, brain fog (problems with memory and concentration), and sleep disturbance with unrefreshing sleep. I also had a host of other symptoms, including shortness of breath, poor balance, dizziness, muscle weakness, headaches, digestive issues, muscle spasms, multiple chemical sensitivities, and probably more.

b. I also had a diagnosis of diastolic heart dysfunction.

My Heart Problem:

When I saw Dr. Brewer in October 2011 — which was my fourteenth office visit with him — the doctor told me that there was good evidence in the cardiology literature that diastolic dysfunction in the heart was caused by mitochondria dysfunction. He also told me that a Texas cardiologist named Peter Langsjoen had recommended CoQ10 for my type of congestive heart failure.

Furthermore, Dr. Brewer told me that there were two kinds of CoQ10: ubiquinone and ubiquinol. He said, in a small study published in late 2008, Dr. Langsjoen had showed that ubiquinol was superior in treating heart patients over the cheaper and more commonly sold ubiquinone. Dr. Langsjoen had also shown that ubiquinol could reverse diastolic heart dysfunction.

Therefore, Dr. Brewer believed, I should be on an aggressive regimen of taking the ubiquinol. He wanted me to start taking the supplement at 200 mg a day for two to four weeks; and after that, I was to work my way up to 200 mg twice daily.

After our office visit, on the 1st of November, I started taking the ubiquinol as suggested by the doctor.

In December, my social worker paid me a visit. She was shocked at how ill I was, and she even told me that she had seen people on their death beds who looked better than I did. She proceeded to get me into in-home hospice care. Based on a letter from my cardiologist, my hospice diagnosis was diastolic heart failure.

On December 25, I added to the ubiquinol the supplement D-ribose, but only when I felt it was needed. It was supposed to be an important player in cellular energy (ATP).

Then, in February 2012, I began experiencing kidney pain. My research on the Internet back then indicated that there was only one common cause of both heart pain and kidney pain: a lack of adequate potassium. Then I remembered that I had once read somewhere that CFS patients were usually low in potassium. So on the 1st of March 2012, I began taking 800 mg of potassium daily. Two weeks later, I added in a magnesium supplement.

At the end of March, I remained extremely ill. Also, my chest pain had become more severe. I was prescribed 2.5 ml of liquid morphine and 5 mg tablets of the opioid oxycodone — to be taken as needed.

For the next several months, my chest pain and my heart proceeded to get worse. Then, surprisingly, my heart actually begun to show some improvement near the end of October.

Finally, in mid-January 2013, one of my hospice nurses came to check me out of hospice. I asked her if many people ever got off of hospice. She said maybe 2%, if that. She also confided in me that when she first became one of my hospice nurses on a Monday during one week that previous September, she thought (to herself) that I was so bad that I wouldn't make it through the upcoming weekend. She said she was glad I had survived.

One concern I had about being discharged from hospice, however, was how I would deal with those heart pain and air hunger episodes that sometimes still got pretty bad. I worried about not being able to continue to take my morphine and oxycodone for those episodes.

Then, through a good friend, I found out who had overseen my hospice treatment and care plan. It was Dr. A., and she also had a family medicine practice in a suburb of Kansas City, Kansas. I made an appointment and went to see her. I told her about my concerns. She asked me if I needed any morphine or opioids at that time. I said, "No." She told me to come back and see her if that situation changed.

I saw Dr. A. a few more times in 2013, but not for obtaining morphine and opioids. As time passed, it was apparent I didn't need to be on those drugs anymore.

However, my chest pain did continue, albeit at a more moderate level, until the 1st of October, 2013, when I started on a antifungal medication prescribed by Dr. Brewer for a toxic mold infection.   Shortly after that, surprisingly, my chest pain improved dramatically.

Chapter One: Toxic Mold

<u>Office Visit #15 with Dr. Brewer on June 28, 2012:</u>

Once Dr. Brewer had reviewed my medical file and my office visit notes, I began recording our visit.

Dr. Brewer: "Let me tell you about an interesting new thing I've gotten into. ... The subject matter is people who have been exposed to toxic mold.

"How I got into this is, I have a young patient that was sent to me for Lyme disease a few years ago. She's in her twenties. I got a phone call in February from her father, and he told me that they had tested their whole family for mold toxins. I believe there were five of them: mom, dad, and three children. And they all tested positive, including this girl who was my patient. I was intrigued by the test, what had transpired and so forth, because I had not heard of this test before.

"Now the reason they pursued this [is that] they have a second home, a summer home in a different state. And apparently last summer, they were there for the whole summer, and they saw evidence of mold in the house. So then in the fall, after they had left, they brought in a mold testing company and had [the house tested for mold]. They knew there was mold there, but they didn't know if it was the kind that would give rise to health consequences.

"Apparently the test results were bad, and they had extensive mold problems, and they had toxic mold in the house. The father said his whole family had been exposed, and maybe it was there the year before and they weren't aware of it.

"So he pursued seeing what testing was available [for the members of his family], and he ended up getting these mold toxin tests done.

"The lab that does this toxic mold testing is located down in Dallas. I had not heard of this lab before February, and I was unaware of this test. I have actually done a fair amount of reading about mold toxins over the last 10 years or so, so I know a fair amount about it. It's not something I've kept up with, every little bit and piece from the literature, and it's not something I read up on regularly. But I was intrigued by this. And I had this girl who was ill, who had the Lyme disease diagnosis, but also now had this toxin thing. And then the whole family tested positive [for the mold toxins].

"So the first thing I did was, I did my due diligence on the lab. What is the test? Is it valid? How long had they been doing it, and what kind of data did they have, etc.? So I did a lot of looking up on the lab; I read their research papers; I called them up and talked to them on the phone; etc. To make a long story short, the lab is excellent. It is a very good laboratory. I pretty much arrived at that conclusion after I had really done quite a bit of due diligence on them.

"So the next thing I did, I started updating my reading and studying on mold illness. [I wanted to know] what new things had been published since I'd last looked at it; what were some of the new findings; etc. So I have done an enormous amount of reading about mold illness and so forth over the last four months. And like I'm doing with you today, I'm discussing [this] with all my chronic illness patients. It was a very interesting spring, to say the least.

"[Now] previously healthy people can probably be divided into a couple of categories. One is people who are allergic to mold, and they will typically have respiratory issues. The common one is sinuses. They'll have chronic sinus problems due to the mold allergies. Then they can have asthma. Those people will react to virtually any mold because they are mold allergic. So any time they're breathing in significant amounts of mold that they're allergic to, it could cause some problems. Indoor mold, outdoor mold, either of them. In fact, many times those people will have more trouble outdoors than indoors.

"Now the other issue, the part that got me into this, is the toxic mold issues. That's a much different problem. Because here we're *not* talking about allergies; we're talking about actual toxins that are produced by certain strains of mold. And these are extremely toxic substances, pound-for-pound probably some of the most toxic substances on earth. Not all molds are toxic; only some molds are toxic.

"The interesting twist to this is that most of the toxic mold problems are found inside of buildings. This is what we call indoor mold problems. The link that ties all these issues together, with the toxic mold and so forth, is usually a water problem with the building. Getting water into the building where it's not supposed to be. So this could be rain water getting into the basement or up in the attic, leaking windows, etc. Or it could be an indoor plumbing problem: a pipe that breaks, a shower problem, dishwasher, washing machine that's got a leak behind it, something like that.

"So what happens is, the mold spores are pretty much [on the] inside of all buildings. And when water gets in there, the spores will germinate and start to grow into mold. Before that, the spores are dormant. But as water comes into contact with them, [the spores] will begin very quickly, in one to two days, to start growing into mold. As the mold grows, it will then begin to produce the toxins. Now these toxins are chemicals, and they get into the air. And in the air they are invisible; you cannot see them and you cannot smell them. So you don't know they're there. So the person is breathing them in, being unaware that they are breathing them in.

"Once they get into the body, they go down into the lungs and rapidly diffuse into the blood stream … and circulate throughout the body. As they circulate throughout the body, they can go anywhere.

"They can affect the kidneys, liver. They can get into the brain and nervous system. They can affect any organ in the body. One of the curious things — and again, these are very dangerous toxins that can create major issues with people's health — one of the interesting things they do that may relate to CFS, Lyme disease, etc. is that they can be significant suppressors of the immune system, including natural killer cells. The natural killer cell thing has been pretty well documented. So the immune system gets significantly screwed up by these toxins, and they can do all kinds of other things too.

"Now the symptoms of toxic mold cases is a lengthy list of symptoms that essentially looks identical to those of CFS, fibromyalgia, chronic Lyme disease, etc. It's a very long list of symptoms … but they're real.

"The association between the symptoms and the mold exposure is a lot of times very tight, where the person says, 'I was completely healthy until I worked in that office building that had mold in it. [Then] I started developing fatigue, and headaches, and brain fog, and pain, and other things. And that all occurred after I worked in that sick building.'

"So, every symptom you have is on the mold list.

"I used to think, prior to the last few months, that if somebody was exposed [to mold] three or four years ago, and they developed some symptoms after the known exposure, [that] if you took them out of that environment, and they're not there any more — they either don't live there anymore, or they don't work in the building that they thought had made them sick, or whatever — if you get them out of that environment, then one would assume that they would clean things out. They would detox, and things would get cleaned up, and the symptoms would resolve. It turns out, that's not true. These toxins can persist for very long periods of time, if not almost indefinitely.

"Now let's turn our attention to the test, because the test is sort of what kind of documents this. The test is a urine test. You simply pee in a cup and mail it to the lab in Dallas. They assay your urine. Now what they're looking for in the urine are the actual toxins themselves. So they're assaying the urine for the toxic chemicals that are produced by molds that grow indoors. The test is extremely accurate; it can measure the toxins down to very, very low levels. It can't quite go to zero, but it gets down very close to zero.

"The test essentially does not have false positives. So if you take healthy people who say, 'I feel fine, and to my knowledge, I have not been exposed to mold,' they would virtually never test positive. On the other hand, if you take known mold exposures — like this family that I was telling you about; and remember, the family was 100%, five out of five positive for mold toxins — so if you take known mold exposures, the hit rate on a positive test is about 90% to 95%. So the test, if somebody has a known exposure, is correct about 95% of the time, which means it only has about 5% false negatives. And it has virtually zero false positives. That's a really good test. So when I get a test result back, I know I have an accurate, reliable result.

"So let's say I test you. You pee in a cup; you send your urine down to Dallas, and we get a result back on you. And it's positive, and it shows mold toxins in the urine. That tells me, without question, that you have mold toxins inside of you. You have to, because your body is trying to rid itself of them in the urine. You're trying to get rid of the toxins in the urine. When we test somebody who's positive, we know that they've got toxic mold inside them.

"The lab in Dallas has a number of cases that they tested where the person was exposed — they have symptoms, and they had a positive urine test — but their exposure was many years ago, and they may not be currently under exposure. So, the toxins are still coming out years down the line, which suggests that they are still getting new toxins into the system.

"That kind of gets to what I call my input/output model. This applies to how I think the model works; and it also applies to treatment, which might be extremely successful. In other words, if this is a big deal — which I think it is — this may be an effective treatment for CFS cases that are chronically mold toxic. And we may be able to reverse the symptoms. So this is a big deal. This is treatable.

"But the treatment, it's critical to understanding what I call the input/output issue. So the output issue is, we're taking somebody that has been documented as having toxins in their urine, and we'll make an assumption that we think those toxins are creating your symptoms. We think that those toxins — these very dangerous toxins that are inside your system — are responsible for at least part, or maybe a lion's share, or possibly all of your symptoms. But [the patients] are actually getting rid of [the mold toxins] every time they go and urinate, and the toxins are going down the toilet. So [the patients] are getting rid of them. So that's the output.

"If there is no input; if there are no new toxins coming into the body … and the output continues, the [patient] will get rid of the toxins and their symptoms will go away. But we have a problem with input. … So what are the input issues? I think there are two that have to be addressed.

"One is external to the body; and the other is internal, inside the body.

"The external one is, are [patients] living in an environment — which in your case would be your apartment — are they living in an environment in which there is mold or toxic mold in that environment? And then every time they're in that environment, they're breathing in more mold toxins.

"I'm not saying that applies to you, and I'm not saying that applies to all my patients. But the point is, if you ignore that piece of it, the patient will never get well as long as they live in that environment. Because that's how they got it in the first place … in their environment. This is an environmental illness.

"So if they're getting [incoming mold toxins from] their environment, they can't win. They're just spinning their wheels. Yes, they're peeing [the mold toxins] out, but they're putting new ones back in every time they're inside that home or apartment or whatever. Or it could also be a work building, if people are still working. So a person needs to give some thought and consideration to their environment. …

"The internal issue applies to where the patients lived and worked in the past. The internal issue is that they may have actually inhaled mold spores into their body … and that they actually have an active mold infection inside their body. Now this could be in a variety of places, but one would think the most likely would be the sinuses, lungs, GI tract, intestines, and so forth. So they may have mold issues internally, inside of their body, and they're internally producing their own toxins. So that's the internal problem.

"So the treatment strategy is to choke off both sources of input. And then again, we've already proven that the patients will get rid of the toxins because they've had a positive urine test. So they will continue to pee them out and get rid of them, and they should eventually be able to clear them out. … [But] one has to address the input. …

"[Now] for those patients who have tested positive for the mold, we're basically using antifungal drugs. … These are oral medications, taken by mouth, that will kill the mold. Those are the ones we're talking about. So for my people who are testing positive, the general thing I'm going with are these antifungal medications.

"[So the thinking is, if you get rid of the actual mold from inside the body,] then the toxin production will stop internally. [So for] the patient, as long as they're not taking it in from their environment, the toxin production will stop. And they'll be able to clear the mold toxins. And they should see significant clinical improvement.

"There may be some herbal preparations and so forth that are effective in treating the mold in the body as well. We don't have as much data about that as we do on the antifungals, but there may be some alternatives to the prescription medications. This is just one example, but it's a good one: oil of oregano. It's an extremely potent antifungal compound. It's been talked a lot about, in the CFS circles, even as a yeast medication or supplement. It will actually kill a number of the molds as well. That's just one example of some natural compounds that might be effective, but they haven't been as well studied as the pharmaceutical ones.

"As of last Friday, 82 of my patients have submitted their urine to the lab in Dallas for the toxin assay, and 72 are positive. [That's] 72 out of 82, so essentially 90%, which is about what the lab gets on mold exposure cases. Now I can talk to the patient, and … most of them can think of some exposure history. But again, their exposures, many of them, were in the past. These are patients who are just starting out from a basic standpoint. The patient is sick, and they have health problems that match up with things like CFS and fibromyalgia.

"So we're kind of going about it backwards, where we're saying, 'Okay, we're taking a sick patient and asking the intuitive question, could this be mold illness?' We're going to roll the dice on this and see if this could be known mold illness. And, in 90%, the roll of the dice came up positive. And remember, the test does not have false positives.

"Now many of them do remember exposure, but it may be in the past. Some of them, we think, have it in their homes at the present time. So it's a mixture of everything, and stories of what's happening in the house is everything you can imagine. I've heard the dishwasher story, the washing machine story, the broken pipe behind the wall, the leaky roof, the leaky basement.

"And remember, you've got to go back, for all intents and purposes, your whole life. Even [to] when you were young. Any known problems with buildings that you lived or worked in, that had a water problem or any known mold exposure.

"My opinion is, if somebody tests positive — and you basically might have a 90% chance of testing positive — we know they have [the mold] in their system. It's probably the reason they're ill, [maybe not a 100% of the reason, but it's] at least a major contributor as to why they're ill. [You have to get rid of the toxic mold from out of your current environment, and you have to get rid of the toxic mold from out of your body], and that's the route to getting better."

Bob: "When I got sick, I was living in Manhattan [Kansas]. And we had flood waters on three sides of the town for several months, and I was always coming down with colds and flu and stuff." Dr. Brewer: "What year was that?" Bob: "That was the same year I got sick, 1993." Dr. Brewer: "Oh, that was the big '93 floods." Bob: "Yes. The doctors tested me for allergies, and I came up as being allergic to mold. Could I have gotten mold exposure through the air because of all the flood waters?"

Dr. Brewer: "Yes, possibly."

Bob: "Also, I was working in a building where they were tearing out what they called the *good asbestos*, whatever that means. [We both laughed at the oxymoron.] I did spend some time working down on those floors where this was going on, and they were tearing a lot of the walls out, so there could have been mold exposure there." Dr. Brewer: "There could have been, because to get at the asbestos, they have to get into the walls and up in the ceilings." … Bob: "So I had two possibilities for mold exposure back then."

Dr. Brewer: "The thing that makes this quite interesting [for you] is … the sequence of events fits." The doctor went on to give me another example of this.

Dr. Brewer: "Most of the mold experts now think that 50% of all mold is not visible [in buildings]."

Bob: "So are you going to have me take this test?" Dr. Brewer: "That's going to be your choice. Because there's a hitch." We both laughed at that. "The hitch is, we're not sure that Medicare's paying for it. It's a $525 test. … So the question is, are you willing to roll the dice on $525? …

"I'd love for you to get the test, because I'll be quite honest and blunt with you, it might be the best $525 you ever spent. [That's] because it might be the answer to what's been wrong with your health all these years. And you say, 'Well, Dr. Brewer, how can you say that?' [And I reply, 'Because] I have 72 reasons, [72 positive mold exposure tests on patients so far], is why I can say that.'"

We discussed that the urine test is a *kit,* and you take the test at home; and that to get a mold test done for your environment at home, it costs around $100 to $300.

Office Visit #16 with Dr. Brewer on December 18, 2012:

Note 1: As of this visit, I had not done anything in regard to testing for mold in my apartment, or in taking the mold toxin urine test from the Dallas Lab. ~~

In my notes for the doctor, I wrote: My fatigue is worse than ever most of the time, and I am sicker than ever much of the time. When I am at my very worst, I don't see how I could be so very ill and still be alive.

Note 2: For the beginning of our office visit, there were two papers referred to:

(1) Regarding the retrovirus seen in CFS patients, this appeared in a paper published by Elaine DeFreitas in the April 1, 1991, issue of the *Proceedings of the National Academy of Sciences* (Vol. 88, Issue 7).   The article was entitled: "Retroviral sequences related to human T-lymphotropic virus type II in patients with chronic fatigue immune dysfunction syndrome." Among the 10 authors listed were: E DeFreitas … P R Cheney, D S Bell … It can be seen on the web site: https://www.pnas.org/content/88/7/2922.

(2) The second paper was published in the Annals of Internal Medicine, 15 January 1992; Vol 116 (2):103-13. The article was entitled: "A Chronic Illness Characterized by Fatigue, Neurologic and Immunologic Disorders, and Active Human Herpesvirus Type 6 Infection." Among the 17 authors listed were: … Paul R. Cheney, MD, PhD; Daniel L. Peterson, MD … Robert C. Gallo, MD … It can be seen on the website: http://www.ncf-net.org/library/ AnnalsofInternalMed92-1106.htm. ~~

First there was a review of my file and my visit notes. Then Dr. Brewer told me that the XMRV retrovirus thing was *zero* now, meaning it had been confirmed that it was a non-entity as a player in CFS.

Bob: "When you read [the book] *Osler's Web*, it seems like it's a foregone conclusion that it's a retrovirus that's involved in

CFS." Dr. Brewer: "Right." Bob: "I mean, Drs. Paul Cheney and Daniel Peterson and David Bell and the researcher Elaine DeFreitas had all worked together, and they had all thought it was a retrovirus.

"There was also a paper put out where there must have been 50 of the world's top virologists who had signed-off on the idea that CFS was most likely caused by the retrovirus discovered by DeFreitas, and that probably HHV-6 played a role in that as well. Dr. Cheney signed it; Dr. Robert Gallo [the co-discoverer of the HIV virus] signed it; there was a whole bunch of people who signed off on that."

Dr. Brewer: "Yes, I'm aware of all that. I've read all that. And I've actually met the author of *Osler's Web*. I know Cheney; I know Peterson; I know Gallo; I've met all the players. I've never met DeFreitas, because she's retired in Florida. She's in poor health. There's some attractiveness to the retrovirus models, but certainly it looks like, if there is any association with a retrovirus, it's not XMRV. [And I've cooled] a little bit on the retroviruses."

This prompted another of our many brief discussions held over the years on the possibility of retrovirus activity in CFS. (Dr. Brewer is quite knowledgeable about retroviruses, and he sees HIV/AIDS patients as well as CFS patients.)

Dr. Brewer: "Now the newest development, which we talked about last time, is the mold stuff. That's turned out to be a pretty big deal. … In my experience, [this is] the most compelling thing I've ever come across. And it's pretty impressive.

"Part of the issue with the mold toxins is that the test is just so darned accurate. The test, basically, is one of the most accurate things we can do. Because we're not testing for antibody, or a virus, or a PCR; we're not doing anything like that at all. We're actually testing for a chemical. So it would be like testing for DDT or dioxin … where the report comes back in parts per billion. … We can detect infinitesimally small amounts of these toxins."

The doctor went on to say how this was important when it came to testing the healthy controls used by the Dallas lab, all of whom had come up *zero* for toxic mold.

Dr. Brewer: "So I have now tested right at 220 patients with the urine/mycotoxin assay from the lab in Dallas, and I have 200 positives. So I've only had 20 negative tests since last February. So we're running right at a 90% positive rate. We are preparing a paper to publish on this, on the first 100 or so that we tested. We've pretty much got the paper finished; we're just trying to figure out which journal to submit it to. They'll be several authors on the paper, including a couple of major mold experts, so we've come a long way on that.

"But in most of my cases, the dots actually connect really nicely. Most of them, over 90%, have some history of mold exposure. Or at least being exposed to a damp, moisture-problem building with or without obvious mold. They all have sort of a standard CFS-type illness, and they have the positive mold toxin assay.

"Now one of the ways this would *not* negate or exclude other issues like EBV, or HHV-6, Lyme disease, etc., including possibly even retroviruses, is that these toxins suppress the immune system. That's not even controversial. We know these mold toxins suppress the immune system; that's been well-published.

"I think the mold toxin thing is a bit of a domino effect. But as I tell people, I think the first domino, and the most important domino, and the ongoing domino, is the mold toxins. But I think there are secondary players in this: viruses; if a person has been exposed to ticks, maybe Lyme disease; etc.

"The other thing, tied-in with your heart and with your other symptoms, is this whole concept of mitochondrial dysfunction. Which is the basis for the [heart/energy] supplements you're on. As you and I have talked about before, there is extensive data about mitochondrial dysfunction in patients with CFS.

"[Dr.] Myhill just published another paper within the last month out of London. It's a follow-up study on her 120 some patients that she found had abnormal energy output stuff, with the ATP work and so forth that they've done. So I think the evidence is pretty overwhelming."

Bob: "Are you talking about the mold toxins now?" Dr. Brewer: "I haven't got there yet, but that's what I'm going to say. You're just one slight step ahead of me. So we have evidence that CFS patients have mitochondrial malfunction. That's nothing new; that's been known for at least a decade, with many studies from all over the world showing evidence of that.

"There's extensive data, for all the toxins, that they're poisons to mitochondria. And I mean extensive. And this will be in our paper. … The mechanism of how these toxins may lead to CFS is their mitochondrial poisons. We're going to have probably at least 15 references in our study.

"[So] the mold toxins absolutely explain mitochondrial malfunction. It would absolutely explain immune malfunction. And then, with the immune malfunction, it would then give you a mechanism why latent infections like EBV and HHV-6 can surface."

In response to a question from me, the doctor said that *toxins* and *poisons* mean the same thing.

We then discussed the mold toxin test, and how it was still $525, and how it was still not covered by Medicare. The doctor said that, instead of 200 positive mold test results, he would have about 350 such positives by now if all his Medicare patients could afford to take the test.

Dr. Brewer: "The other question, of course, that we're dealing with in all of this is, 'How to treat this?' We're working at it from two different angles. One is trying to enhance the elimination of the mold toxins out of the body, and [the other one is] to prevent new toxins from coming in."

The doctor went on to talk again about living environments that contain toxic mold, and how his patients could not get better as long as they continued to stay in those types of environments.

"The other issue is whether they have any mold inside their body … that could be producing toxins internally."

"[So] we've had several patients get completely well. But it's not everybody. And some of the medicines that are working for patient A are not working for patients B, C, and D. So right now it's not one size fits all for the treatments. But I do think we know what the highway looks like on the treatments. It's a clear-cut highway."

Bob: "What are you using to treat people?" Dr. Brewer: "The antifungals; we're using these oral antifungals." Here the doctor named both of the drugs. "The problem is, both of those can have side effects, and both of them are expensive."

Dr. Brewer went on to say the results he'd seen so far with his patients on these drugs had been one third, one third, one third. About one third had seen substantial or incredibly dramatic improvement, or had gotten completely well; about one third had seen no change at all; and about one third had experienced side-effects.

The doctor then talked about some of the side effects seen with the oral antifungal use; and he also went on to give a specific example of a patient who had almost completely recovered her health before the drug's side effects became too intolerable. At that point, she was switched over to taking the other of the two antifungal drugs the doctor had been using.

Dr. Brewer: "There's a 90% chance you're a mold case, just based on statistics. I've tested 220 people for the toxic mold, and 200 of them are positive. And the test is virtually never wrong. So there is a 90% chance that you're a mold case. So you're saying, I can't really afford the drugs — actually, I won't give them to you anyway, unless you have a positive test, I can't do that — but a simple little thing you can make sure of is that you're not living in a moldy environment. And there is some testing that can be done and so forth. [But] if you're in a moldy environment, you will remain ill."

The doctor went on to discuss mold in apartments, homes, and other buildings; and the different kinds of mold testing available for those environments.

Bob: "How have patients done using oregano for treatment?" Dr. Brewer: "It's been mixed."

Bob: "Well, you've had a pretty high number of patients test positive for the mold, 90%." Dr. Brewer: "I thought so. And the test is so good. If we were still doing a PCR test, for some virus or something like that … then are we going down another XMRV road? But this is a totally different test. This is testing for a chemical. … That's what so cool about the test; it's so accurate."

<u>Office Visit #17 with Dr. Brewer on June 24, 2013:</u>

After a review of my file and my visit notes, in response to a question from me, Dr. Brewer said: "Mold and fungus mean the same thing." He then went on to speak about the purpose of mold in life and what functions the mold served. "But only a few of the molds make toxins," he said. And in humans, "the mold can be poisonous to us. … [The mold can] poison the mitochondria.

"Our point is, there's very little question, based on the literature that's now been published over the last 10 or 15 years … that what CFS patients have, among other things, is they have mitochondria dysfunction. Their mitochondria don't work right. And there's no question whatsoever that mold toxins are toxic to mitochondria. So now we're saying, we find mold toxins in 93% of CFS cases, is it not the basis of their illness?"

The doctor said that through this past week, his patients who had tested positive for the toxic mold toxins had grown to 255 positives; and that, overall, his patients were still running 90% to 95% in testing positive for the mold.

The doctor went on to mention that a number of his patients could recall living in some kind of housing that had mold present back when they first got sick. And even though most of these patients had long since been removed from that situation into non-moldy housing, they had remained sick; and they had also tested positive for mold toxins. So, Dr. Brewer said: "There is only one conclusion we can come to. … [These patients] actually have the mold inside their bodies. …

"So my current thinking is, all of you have toxic-producing mold inside your body. So then the question is, where is it and how do we get rid of it? … If you can can get rid of the mold toxins, that patient will presumably regain health … [or at least] it would get rid of the symptoms directly related to CFS.

"Since these are mitochondrial toxins, they could easily be leading to diastolic dysfunction. They could be leading to some of the heart issues. These are known liver toxins … and if you were to test toxin positive, is there a role for the toxins in the liver? Maybe. We don't know." Bob: "I do have some liver damage, and something's caused that." …

Dr. Brewer: "So the question is — in these patients not being currently exposed externally — if we can get rid of the mold out their body, their toxin levels should drop over time. Hopefully drop down close to that zero mark, which is where those healthy people are. And then they would regain health. So again, the question is, where is the mold inside the body and how do we get rid of it?

"So the newest hypothesis we have … Again, when I call these hypotheses, these are based on extensive amounts, and I do mean extensive amounts, of published literature. These aren't us just guessing. What we're saying is, we're trying to connect dots, and the dots would seem to connect through what's already been published in the literature. So we think the main place [the toxic mold is] localized inside the body is inside the patients' sinuses.

Bob (stunned): "Really?"

This was followed by us talking over each other briefly, before I went quiet and let the doctor continue.

"All this stuff I'm telling you today is pretty new; not stuff we're quoting in the literature, but this kind of sinus hypothesis. We've only come up with this in about the last three months.

"So the concept is, you breathe in the mold spores out of a toxic building; they get inside your sinuses, and the mold is going to stay in there the rest of your life. And unless we diminish those levels, or get rid of it, then we lose the ball game in terms of the CFS. That's my current strategy, my current hypothesis.

"Now, why do we think the sinuses?" He said he was currently writing a paper on this. "A lot of the original data that steers us in that direction came from the Ear, Nose and Throat [ENT] group at the Mayo Clinic when they were studying chronic sinus patients.

"These were people who have chronic sinus problems, chronic sinusitis. So Mayo did a study where they went up into people's noses and sinuses with a scope and looked around; looked for inflammation and so forth. And then they took cultures for mold and fungus out of their sinuses.

"What they found is that everybody has mold and fungus in their sinuses, including normal healthy people. [That] kind of makes sense, because you're breathing air. You walk out today, there's going to be quite a bit of mold spores in the air. Now it's not toxic mold spores; those are just regular outdoor mold spores. So it's not surprising that some of those spores are going to end up landing in one's sinuses and just staying there.

"All of us have mold and fungus in our nose and sinuses. For most folks, that's going to be standard outdoor mold that is innocuous and doesn't produce toxins. Doesn't really cause any problems. The difference between chronic sinus patients and a normal healthy person — because they have the same kinds of mold in their sinuses — is that the chronic sinus patient is allergic to mold. … We've simply taken that a step further and say that people with CFS have toxic mold in their sinuses.

"So instead of being allergic to the mold, the species of mold that are in their sinuses — and they could have both; some of these patients have both — but instead of just being flatly allergic to it, the mold that's in [the sinuses of CFS patients] has the capacity to produce toxins. And we think those toxins get absorbed through the wall of the sinuses; cross right into the blood stream; circulate through the blood stream 24/7, 365; and some it comes out in the urine every day. So there's basically an internal factory."

Bob: "Where's it start? In the sinuses? The mold's in the sinuses?" Dr. Brewer: "And it introduces the toxins, and they're small chemicals." … Bob: "You're breathing these chemicals in?" Dr. Brewer: "No, the chemicals are produced internally. But initially you breathe it in.

"Let's say you were in a moldy toxic house 20 years ago. Initially you breathe it in. Then the actual mold gets in the sinuses. The mold is what produces the toxins. Remember, [the toxins are] chemicals. [These] chemicals are very small molecules so they will cross membranes. They can go right into your brain; they can go right across your sinuses into the blood stream; they can go inside of cells; [they] can go throughout your body."

Bob: "These are the spores or the toxins?" Dr. Brewer: "The toxins." Bob: "But they're awfully small, so that's why you call them micro-toxins?" Dr. Brewer: "No, *myco* means mold. It's not 'micro,' it's m-y-c-o. The word *myco* means mold or fungus. Mold toxin and mycotoxin are the same thing.

"So what we're saying is, the mold spores and so forth are inside your sinuses; those produce the chemicals; the chemicals get into your blood stream and could go directly into your brain, and circulate through your system, and your body tries to get rid of them. Which it does. Because remember (inaudible) the urine test; it's coming out in the urine. But the reason the body can't get rid of all of this is, because there is an internal factory."

Bob: "And that factory is located in the sinuses?"

Dr. Brewer: "That's what we think; that's our hypothesis. If that's true, then, we should direct our treatment at the sinuses. Which then our newest treatment is using direct intranasal antibiotics and antifungals that we're spraying through the nose, to try to kill the mold and fungus out of the sinuses by direct intranasal (inaudible)."

Bob: "So before you were using oral drugs? And weren't those pretty expensive? And weren't some people having some serious side effects?"

Dr. Brewer: "That is correct. So now we're going to an intranasal approach, which is not expensive [and which] does not have any systemic side effects. Now we are seeing some interesting die-off reactions, where we're putting people on intranasal antifungals, and they actually feel a little bit worse for a week or two because of the die-off reaction.

"Now the intranasal thing is very new. We've only been doing that about six weeks, so I can't give you much feedback." Bob: "What's it called?" Dr. Brewer: "All we're doing is spraying an antifungal up the nose. It's intranasal … intranasal delivery, if you will, of antifungals. So these are not identical to the ones we were giving in pills, but similar. And we're using this pharmacy in California that's using this [atomizer] device to deliver them up into the nose and sinuses."

Bob: "How expensive is this?" Dr. Brewer: "Not very expensive." Bob: "That's progress." Dr. Brewer: " What's your prescription coverage? Do you have Medicare Part D?" Bob: "Yes." Dr. Brewer: "Some of the Medicare Part D is paying for it. It's not terribly expensive, because all the drugs are generic.

And we're still learning what cocktail works the best, combining a couple of different sprays and so forth."

So I went ahead and asked how I would go about getting my apartment checked for toxic mold. The doctor said I could ask my apartment management to check my apartment for mold, or I could hire somebody myself to do it. At this point, the doctor gave me the name of just such a testing company to call and use in Lawrence, Kansas, where I lived. He said they would do a good job with the mold testing.

Bob: "But first I would do the urine test, to see if I had the mold?" Dr. Brewer: "Yes, yes, right. And that's problematic too, because the urine test is still $525, and Medicare doesn't pay for it. That's the bad news."

A good deal of inaudible talk followed, as there was construction noise in the background.

Dr. Brewer: "I'm pretty convinced that the mold and mold toxins are a massive player in your illness. I don't know if they're the only player, but I believe they are the major player."

The doctor then said that people often asked him how his paper had been received. Dr. Brewer: "I'd say about 80% has been very positive. There's been about 20% that's been negative, with people saying that's so silly, this is too simple, etc. ...

"Let's face it here. We're throwing a whole new monkey wrench into CFS. What I'm saying is, about 80% of people have liked the monkey wrench and about 20% have not."

A lot of miscellaneous talk followed before we returned to the issue of the mold and mold toxins.

Dr. Brewer: "Our whole thing with mold and mold toxins is, we have shown a striking correlation. Is it cause and effect? Well, if it is, then you ought to be able … to take somebody with elevated mold toxins; and take [those mold toxin levels down] to zero; and [then see the patient] get well. [And] I've already had several get well … fully recovered.

"Now I've had that happen in a few patients on the oral antifungals. I saw a guy about a month ago that went from bedridden to well in three months. … I've had several get fully recovered. I've had several that got fully recovered, and we took them off the antifungal, and they relapsed. What happened? Did we get rid of all of it? I'm telling you what, this getting rid it out of the sinuses is not going to be easy. … [But] it's not impossible. It's very doable." …

But, he said, if you had toxic mold in your sinuses, "I guarantee you this. It will continue to produce toxins for the rest of your life."

So I asked for a test kit for the mold toxins, which he gave me. You pay for the test with a credit card when it's sent in.

My liver problem was mentioned. Dr. Brewer: "It's not even controversial that these mold toxins are mitochondrial toxins. That's not even controversial. It's extensively published. [So] this could be affecting your liver. This could be affecting your heart. This could have multiple effects."

Bob: "Could these mold toxins attack the detox enzymes in your liver?" Dr. Brewer: "Yes, and then you might not be able to detox." …

As to the issue of mold and mold toxins, Dr. Brewer said: "I'm pretty optimistic. In doing CFS for almost 30 years now, this is the most amazing thing I've ever come across."

I then asked him about the approximate 7% of his CFS patients that didn't test positive for mold toxicity. The doctor said half of those patients had mold readings very close, but just under, the cut off point they used for diagnosing infection. The other half of those patients were not very sick, and indeed most of them were still working. So it was understandable that they didn't test positive for mold infection. Otherwise they would have been more ill, like those patients testing positive.

When I asked the doctor about the R-Nase L enzyme that I had believed for so long was said to be what attacked our mitochondria, the doctor said that the R-Nase L stuff had been fully discredited. But he said he didn't have time to go into detail on that.

Note: On the website https://www.voiceamerica.com there used to be an interview of Dr. Joseph Brewer by Dr. Neil Nathan dated May 5, 2015. In this interview, Dr. Nathan also talked about the Mayo Clinic study that Dr. Brewer had mentioned to me, saying the information on that study came from a paper published by Mayo in the 1990s.

Before that paper, doctors used to think that chronic sinus infection was mostly bacterial in origin. However, in their study, Mayo found that a large percentage of patients they treated for chronic sinus infection with antibiotics over a long period of time didn't improve.   However, when Mayo began treating these unimproved patients for mold, they did improve.

Dr. Nathan said this had brought about a change in his and Dr. Brewer's thinking, as they began to think that toxic mold was a much bigger player in CFS than they had initially thought. Then Dr. Brewer had built on this information to create his antifungal treatment protocol.

Dr. Brewer said, from that paper, *we* just connected the dots. This meant they now believed that the toxic mold in the sinuses of his CFS patients should respond to an antifungal therapy just as well as the patients had done in the Mayo study. From this belief, Dr. Brewer moved on to treating his CFS patients for toxic mold.

While I couldn't find the specific Mayo paper referred to, I did find several articles on the Internet, dated 1999, about a Mayo Clinic study linking mold and chronic sinusitis. You can see one such article at: https://www.sciencedaily.com/releases/1999/09/990910080344.htm. ~~

Chapter Two: Mold Testing/Meds/Doctors

<u>The Process of Mycotoxin/Home Environment Testing:</u>

(1) First you have to be tested to see if you are infected with the toxic mold. This is done though a RealTime Labs test called a *Mycotoxin Panel,* and it is a urine test that tests for four toxic mold toxins that can be produced by one or more toxic molds. Those four mycotoxins are: ochratoxin, aflatoxin, gliotoxin, and trichothecene (which comes from a variety of molds, including Stachybotrys — or *black mold*).

The *Mycotoxin Panel* is ordered for you by your doctor from: RealTime Labs, 4100 Fairway Drive, Carrollton, Texas, 75010. See them at: http://www.realtimelab.com/.

Originally you had to pay for this test out-of-pocket, but in 2015 most private insurance began to cover this testing; and in early 2016, Medicare also began paying for these tests.

Because most CFS patients are low on glutathione, this can be problematic with the accuracy of the mycotoxin testing. This is because glutathione is important in detoxing the mold toxins out of the body through the urine. So in order to get a more accurate test result on the mycotoxin levels in the body, doctors will often have their CFS patients take a substantial dose of glutathione two times a day for a week. (I've seen 500 mg of glutathione as the suggested dosage to be used twice daily, if the patient can tolerate it.)

Doing this protocol will increase the patient's mycotoxin output in the urine and present a truer picture for any possible mold infection. Then, on the eighth day, patients will take their urine sample and send it in to RealTime Labs, and this way the urine test will pick up patients who might otherwise not test positive for mold.

One doctor who was treating his patients for mold said that, with adding in the glutathione supplementation with his CFS patients *after* their initial mycotoxin testing, he had picked up a dozen positive reports for mycotoxins that had been missed in their earlier testing.

Prior to doctors having their patients take glutathione before their mycotoxin testing, some doctors would have their patients take a sauna from 10 to 30 minutes beforehand, depending on their tolerance. Then the patient would wait a half hour before taking the urine sample for the RealTime Labs test.

From my office visit in July 2016, I had two questions for Dr. Brewer: **Q** (question from me). If someone's mold test falls in the *equivocal* range for infection, is that enough grounds to treat them for a mold infection? **A** (answer from Dr. Brewer). "Yes."

Q. If someone's initial test for any toxic mold infection is negative; and they take glutathione daily for two weeks, or they do a sauna 30 minutes before drawing their urine sample for the mold testing, and the test comes back positive for toxic mold in the second test, is that result valid? **A.** "Yes."

(2) About 10 days after submitting my urine sample to RealTime Labs in mid-June 2013, I received back my *Mycotoxin Panel.* (Back then, they only tested for three mycotoxins; the gliotoxin testing was added to the testing results beginning on February 1, 2016.)

My test showed I had tested positive for two of the three mycotoxins, and those were the ochratoxin and the trichothecene.

After I received my positive mycotoxin test result, Dr. Brewer next had me test my apartment for mold, to insure that I wasn't still being exposed to mold toxins. This he required before he would treat me with any antifungal medication.

I contacted an environmental engineer. He said he would charge me $300 to come out and test my apartment for mold. He also told me that I could buy mold test kits on my own that were very good at mold detection, and that's what he recommended I do for my apartment testing.

So I purchased, over the Internet, the mold test kit that the environmental engineer had recommended to me. It cost $50. I took a 24 hour sample from the stuff that accumulated on my air conditioning and heating unit's air filter, which was to show all of the mold spores circulating inside my apartment's air. My apartment's mold test was *negative* for continuing mold exposure.

The test kit I used came out of Overland Park, Kansas. It was later sold on Amazon for $30, but it doesn't appear to be available any longer. Still, there are many such test kits available on Amazon.

(3) In September 2013, after I had told Dr. Brewer that my apartment had tested negative for mold, he put me on an intranasal antifungal medication called itraconazole.

While Dr. Brewer waits to prescribe an antifungal until after he's sure one's living environment is clear of mold exposure, CFS specialist Dr. Neil Nathan said he goes ahead and prescribes an antifungal right away for his mold patients to take. This is because the antifungal medication can generate some relief where there are circumstances holding back a patient from immediately moving out and away from a moldy environment.

Note: On the RealTime Labs website, it has a section for "International Testing." The two that stood out to me were (a) In the UK: Regenerus Laboratories Limited, Aero 14, Kings Mill Lane, Redhill, Surrey, RH1 5JY, United Kingdom, Tel: +44 (0) 2037500870, Email: info@regeneruslabs.com, and (b) in Australia: NutriPATH, PO Box 442, ASHBURTON, VIC, 3147, Australia, Phone 1300 688 522 (within Australia) or +61 3 9880 2900 (international), Email: info@nutripath.com.au. ~~

The Antifungal Medications Used by Dr. Brewer:

Note: Mold in the nasal passages is protected by a layer of biofilm that must be broken through for any antifungal to be effective. This was discussed at my next office visit. ~~

In 2012, Dr. Brewer had started out treating his patients with oral antifungals.

By mid-2013, he had moved on to using either of two intranasal antifungal drugs, itraconazole or amphotericin B. These were used with the biofilm buster EDTA. By mid-2014, Dr. Brewer had additionally begun using the intranasal antifungal nystatin, also with the EDTA.

(While the other drugs are now taken through the use of a pump sprayer, the nystatin is different. According to an update from Dr. Brewer in January 2015, and using an atomizer, you take the EDTA first; and then, 30 to 60 minutes later, you take the nystatin.)

By mid-2017, the doctor had changed his two original antifungals over to BEG+amphotericin and BEG+itraconazole. These nasal antifungals, along with the EDTA and two antibiotics, come in a pre-mixed nasal spray.

Near the beginning of 2018, Dr. Brewer additionally started treating his patients with the intranasal antifungal colloidal silver. This also comes in a pre-mixed nasal spray, and it contains two biofilm busters, the EDTA and also Mucolox.

Dr. Brewer initially worked with the ASL compounding pharmacy in California to develop his intranasal antifungal and ETDA treatment protocol, as well as for choosing his original intranasal delivery device, which was the NasaTouch atomizer.

The ASL pharmacy is now Imprimis Rx, and their website is at: https://www.imprimisrx.com. Also, the Park Compounding Pharmacy at https://www.parkcompounding.com/compoundcategories/ear-nose-and-throat/ appears to carry some intranasal antifungal medicines. Additionally, the colloidal silver is ordered from: https://pdlabsrx.com.

As for the NasaTouch atomizer, it appears that it is no longer being manufactured, and instead it seems to have been replaced by the Rhino Clear Sprint atomizer.

Note: PD Labs is now operating in the UK as: Compounding Chemists, (+44) 20 3773 2729, hello@pdlabs.co.uk. ~~

<u>Finding a Toxic Mold Health Care practitioner:</u>
You can use the mold lab testing companies to find a mold and mycotoxin health care practitioner:

<u>RealTime Lab:</u>
You can find a health care practitioner, who uses RealTime Lab and specializes in mold and mycotoxin treatment, by area at: https://realtimelab.com/find-a-provider/

Once on this website, it asks you for an order number. I'm guessing that order number comes from ordering a test on their website. The lab told me, if you didn't have an order number, to use "385194." Then they only show you providers within a 25 mile radius, so if you're out in the country, you may have to use a zip code from the nearest big city to find the closest toxic mold practitioners available to you.

Mosaic Diagnostics:
This was formerly known as the Great Plains Laboratory. You can find a health care practitioner, who uses Mosaic Diagnostics toxic mold testing, by going to: https://mosaicdx.com/find-a-practitioner/.

Environmental Doctors:
American Academy of Environmental Medicine at: https://www.aaemonline.org/find-a-practitioner/.

International Society for Environmentally Acquired Illness (ISEAI) at: https://iseai.org/find-a-professional/. However, I didn't see any medical professionals come up in a search of two large cities; instead, one might have better luck on the right side of the webpage under "Medical Professionals."

Robert Roy

<u>Other:</u>

I've been told that the list of doctors who treat for mold infection on the websites shown below are woefully out-of-date, but they're lists I thought I should share anyway, for whatever they may be worth.

Mold Doctors, Environmental Specialists & Clinics
http://www.presenting.net/sbs/molddoctors.html.

Paradigm Change
Mold Illness Practitioners:
https://paradigmchange.me/practitioners/.

Mold-Survivor.com Doctors List - Physician Locator SearchTool:
https://www.mold-survivor.com/DrLists/?state=CA.

(While this website is for California, at the top of the website you can change to any state to search for a mold doctor.)

Surviving Mold
List of Certified Physicians-Shoemaker Protocol:
https://www.survivingmold.com/shoemaker-protocol/Certified-Physicians-Shoemaker-Protocol.

I've read several comments made by people who were successfully treated for mold infection under the Shoemaker protocol, so I have included this website here.

Chapter Three: More Office Visits/Mold

<u>Office Visit #18 with Dr. Brewer on December 19, 2013:</u>

Note: By the time of this visit, I had been taking the nasal antifungal itraconazole at one dose every three days over the past 80 days. ~~

In my notes for the doctor, I wrote: I remain very ill, with and without the antifungal medicine. I am almost totally bedridden, and I am sleeping very little (less than four hours a night). However, my chest pain stopped almost immediately and has not returned.

The doctor began by reviewing my file and my notes since my last visit, including my experience with the itraconazole. We discussed how my health was not good: I felt horrible all over, "like my whole body was turning on itself"; my fatigue was worse, and so was my sleep. Moreover, any improvements I had from the antifungal came in the first month that I was on the drug. Then I had called the doctor's office on November 8, because I was feeling so bad, and I was told then to cut back on my itraconazole use from daily to three times a week.

Dr. Brewer: "Let me review with you the umbrella of what we've seen with people on the intranasal program. You know, in general. …

"First of all, what we think is going on in your nose and sinuses is that there's mold and fungus in there. It's probably embedded in a layer of biofilm, which is this kind of gooey, almost mucus-like substance that is produced by the fungus. In other words, it's a protective layer that the fungus — fungus and mold mean the same thing — it encompasses the mold and fungus. … It protects [the mold] from your immune cells getting to it, and also probably makes it much more difficult for the antifungals to get into it and kill it. …

"We've spent an enormous amount of time looking at this whole concept: the sinuses, and the biofilm, and all that. And we've studied the literature, reviewed the literature on that; and we've written a second paper that just got accepted for publication this week. It's not out yet because we have to do some of the final tweaking of it. But it's basically been accepted, and it will be published in that same journal *Toxins* online. It will probably be available within the next three to four weeks online. …

"So a lot of this background stuff I'm telling you about, biofilm and so forth, we got from researching the literature. So the treatment strategy is basically, largely aimed at two aspects of it. The first one is to break up the biofilm, and that's what the chelating [agent] is to do, is basically what we call the biofilm-buster. And then the [second one is the] itraconazole; it is an antifungal, and it is to kill the fungus. … What we're trying to do is, we're trying to break up the biofilm and kill the fungus. So the two workhorses in your regimen are the chelating [agent] and the itraconazole."

Dr. Brewer went on to discuss how he was getting away from the use of a steroid in his antifungal treatments. He had been using a steroid to try and keep the nose opened up, so the antifungal medicine got into the nasal passages better, but so far he'd found the steroid use to be a mixed bag with his patients. That meant, in the patients taking the steroid: some felt worse, some found it helpful, and some didn't notice anything at all.

Dr. Brewer: "Now this is important. … There's two antifungals that we use. There's only two antifungals that are available right now through ASL. … One is the itraconazole that you're on. The other one is an antifungal called amphotericin. … It's an old, old antifungal that we sometimes use in the hospital intravenously. It's got quite a bit of toxicity, if you use an IV, like [inaudible] kidney toxicity and stuff like that. There isn't any toxicity if you use it nasally, because none of it gets into your body. …

"We probably have, so far, about 175 of you who are doing the intranasal thing. Probably, I'm guessing about two thirds or so, maybe even three fourths, are doing the amphotericin; and then the other third or so are doing the Itraconazol. So it's bit of a mix. … We think they probably work about equally.

"There's a couple of upsides [to the] amphotericin. It's been used more, over the last 10 years, for sinus fungal infections. If you're going to use an intranasal agent for fungal infections of the sinuses, in some of the studies done by Mayo and others, they largely used amphotericin in their studies. And it's also cheaper, because it's an old, generic drug.

"The downside of amphotericin is that it causes quite a bit of nasal irritation and burning. That's due to the chemical nature of the drug itself. It's kind of acidic, so the nose doesn't really like it. The nose feels kind of burning and irritated, and sometimes they get kind of a runny nose. We've had a few people that have had nose bleeds and sinus congestion, that kind of thing. That's the main downside. We do not get very much nasal irritation with the itraconazole.

"On the amphotericin, which again we've used in at least two thirds of cases, we see two negatives. One I've already told you about: that's what I call nasal irritation and burning. And if that gets too harsh or intense with a patient, what we do is, we just back the dose down. …

"Now the other thing we've seen, with either of the agents, is a die-off reaction, or basically the Herxheimer-type reaction. So what's happening there is, when the mold and fungus dies, it releases extra toxin into the body, and which will get into your circulation, and it has to get out of your body. And you're going to feel worse until it gets out of your body." …

Bob: "Does that pass out through the kidneys?" Dr. Brewer: "Yes, it does pass out in your kidneys. ... We don't see the die-off reaction [in everybody]. I would say about half of the patients complain of it, and about half of them don't. The ones that do complain of it ... it varies from mild to severe. In some of them, it's been pretty mild, and they haven't noticed too much. The half that has complained about it, that are worse, they just feel crummy on it. And the most common symptom is fatigue, when they feel worse. Now there could be headaches and other things, but fatigue's the most common thing we see.

"Now with the die-off reaction, what we do there is ... we back down the dose. ... If we think it's a die-off reaction, we basically do the same thing that we do with the nasal burning. [We have them] take it less often. Don't take it everyday; take it every other day, or every third day, or that sort of thing. ...

"We've seen the die-off reaction with both agents, both the itraconazole and the amphotericin. ... [When] we see the die-off reaction, we see it early on. We see it within the first week.

"Now I will say I've had probably three or four patients that didn't notice anything the first two or three days, maybe four or five days. So I've had a handful of patients who said, 'Boy, it went really smoothly for that first two or three days, and then, wow, I started feeling really crummy.'

"[So] maybe it took a few days for that biofilm to start breaking up. ... It's kind of a gel-like substance. ... It starts breaking apart, then the antifungal's penetrating deeper. So you can almost visualize that happening."

With me, I didn't feel any die-off until I'd been on the itraconazole for two months. Dr. Brewer thought that was very odd. Then the doctor spent some time making a comparison of the amphotericin to the itraconazole: the reactions he'd seen in his patients to the drugs, and each of the drugs' negative side effects.

Then the doctor told me that, based on my poor reaction so far to the itraconazole, he wanted to switch me over to the amphotericin. He did mention that, with the amphotericin, "you could get the nasal burning. But we've had to deal with that in over a hundred patients, so [we're used] to dealing with that."

When I told the doctor I had just started on a new prescription of the itraconazole, he said we could make the switch to the amphotericin when my current antifungal prescription ran out, provided I wasn't feeling any better by then.

Then Dr. Brewer said: "Now here's the flip side. So I've told you all the negative stuff, okay. Now I'm going to tell you the positive side. People are getting well right and left on this thing. It works. ... I've had itraconazole patients get well; I've had itraconazole patients improve, some of which, as I've just mentioned, are dramatic. And I've had amphotericin patients improve, and some are dramatic and get well.

"I saw a lady Monday of this week. ... She obviously feels terrible every time I see her. She's kind of a stoic lady that doesn't talk a lot. She's kind of a quiet, unassuming lady. So, I had started her [on the nasal antifungal] in June, and I said, 'So did you start on the nasal thing?' She said, 'Yes, I'm still doing it just like you had prescribed.' And I said, 'So how are you doing on it?' Now this is a quote. She said, 'Oh, I'm well.' End of quote. So I paused for a moment, and I said, 'Come again.' And she goes, 'Oh, I feel great. I think I'm back to normal.' She's been on it since June.

"Now she was on amphotericin, but I've heard similar stories with itraconazole. She did get some of the nasal burning, so she kind of cut back on it. I had originally started her on twice a day. Then we cut back to once a day. And now, she either does it once a day or every other day. She's gone off all her pain medication; her energy levels are great; she's sleeping great.

"I've got about 15 patients like that. And again, to repeat, some of those have been itraconazole cases [and] some of them have been amphotericin cases. But I've got about 15 patients who have essentially gotten well. And I have about 70 patients who are improved."

Bob: "How many of your patients have tested positive for the fungals?" Dr. Brewer: "About 300. That's 300 out of 325. ... I think that's around 95%."

Bob: "And the people that have gotten well, is this a group of people who have been sick as long as I have, 20 years?" Dr. Brewer: "Yes. I have one lady, this is my coolest case, one lady started in June. She's been sick since 1992, 20 years. Her symptoms are very similar to yours; maybe she doesn't have chest pain and that sort of thing. … But she's had fatigue, and brain fog, and all that. She started in June; started feeling really good by July and August. We talked with her in September; she was basically back to normal health by September. So we got her to repeat the urine assay, and the toxins were virtually gone. That's what's really cool about that case.

"Now with you, you had two of the toxins that were elevated. She had all three of them elevated, and her levels were higher than yours. Two of the levels went to zero, and the third one had dropped by 80%. That was from June to late September, we might as well say October 1. … That would be four months, and her toxins essentially almost disappeared.

"We've had four patients who've done really good, and we've repeated the assay, and in all four, the levels have dramatically dropped. That's incredibly encouraging … The question is, the endgame is, we want you to feel better. But the question is, are we affecting the toxin level in your body? And it appears that we are, in a dramatic fashion." …

I asked the doctor, if a patient was allergic to mold like I was, did that make your illness worse? Dr. Brewer: "I think the answer to that is, 'yes.' I think if you're allergic to mold, it makes this worse. Because I get a lot of people who are allergic to mold. Like if they get around mold; if they go visit someone's house and [there's] mold in it, they feel worse. I do think the mold allergy makes it worse." …

Dr. Brewer: "Mold has been talked about as a possible link with CFS in the past. This isn't the first time it's been talked about." Bob (incredulous): "Really?" Dr. Brewer: "But I think the key is, as I mentioned a few minutes ago, the test. I think having that accurate test, it's a game changer. We can even use it as a tool to confirm the patient's getting better. If the patient says, 'Well, Doc, I'm really feeling good,' then we can actually repeat the test. By the way, on the repeat test, the cost drops to $199. ... So I think the test has been huge.

"Now what I tell a lot of people is, I believe this to be, if not *a* key player, *the* key player with CFS. But there's other players, other things than mold ... [like] the immune system, hormones, and possibly viruses like EBV and HHV-6. And in some patients, Lyme disease, etc.

"So I think what happens is, that the mold toxins are the first domino that falls. And then that tips other dominos over, like the immune system, when your immune system goes south. [Then] EBV kicks up, and HHV-6 can kick up, and Lyme can kick up, and you may be more susceptible to things like sinus infections and so forth. And then the hormones go off, and so on and so forth.

"The paper that we published, if you read it real closely, we go to some lengths to discuss that we think the mold toxins are highly toxic to mitochondria. And of course sick mitochondria have been a key piece in CFS."

Bob: "I saw that on the Internet. I also saw that the black mold attacks the heart and liver." Dr. Brewer: "Yes. And kidneys." …

We then reviewed the game plan for me going forward, mostly covering what I would do if, at some point, I did go on the intranasal amphotericin.

Dr. Brewer: "But I tell you, I'm very optimistic. I tell people, this has not been easy. There's been a lot of road bumps, I mean with this nasal burning and the die-off. I mean, I've had several that have nose bleeds; they get irritated in their nose, and they have nose bleeds. … So there's been issues."

We discussed again switching me over to the amphotericin, but at a low dose.

Dr. Brewer: "But the flip side of it is, when you see a person like I saw on Monday of this week, it is jaw-dropping." He then continued to talk about his visit with this lady who was so blasé about getting well.

After some more discussion, Dr. Brewer said: "You're mind's doing pretty well." Bob: "Sometimes." We both laughed at that.

We ended by discussing how suddenly I was doing better with my heart issues and how that seemed to be encouraging.

<u>The First Two Published Papers on Mold by Dr. Brewer et al.:</u>
(1) http://www.mdpi.com/2072-6651/5/4/605. Published 11 April 2013. "Detection of Mycotoxins in Patients with Chronic Fatigue Syndrome" by Joseph H. Brewer, Jack D. Thrasher,

David D. Straus, Roberta A. Madison, and Dennis Hooper. It was published in *Toxins* — "an international, peer-reviewed open access journal which provides an advanced forum for studies related to toxins and toxicology."

(2) http://www.mdpi.com/2072-6651/6/1/66. Published 24 December 2013. "Chronic Illness Associated with Mold and Mycotoxins: Is Naso-Sinus Fungal Biofilm the Culprit?" by Joseph H. Brewer, Jack D. Thrasher, and Dennis Hooper. It was also published in the *Toxins* journal.

Two Early Doctors Testing Their Patients for Mold:
(1) Dr. Brewer told me that in February 2014 he had received an email from Dr. Paul Cheney. (Dr. Cheney then was one of the most respected CFS doctors in America, if not the world.)

According to Dr. Brewer, Dr. Cheney said in his email that he was excited by Dr. Brewer's two published articles on toxic mold in CFS; and that Dr. Cheney had started testing his own CFS patients for mycotoxins, and so far — just like with Dr. Brewer — Dr. Cheney's mold toxin testing was running over 90% positive.

Dr. Chency's last medical practice had been in Asheville, North Carolina. Dr. Cheney had retired in or about 2017, and he passed away in 2021.

Note: Dr. Paul Cheney was involved in what would become known as the "Lake Tahoe Outbreak" of an infectious disease (which was later labeled by the CDC as CFS) in Incline Village, Nevada, in 1984. Incline village is located on the rim of Lake Tahoe. Dr. Cheney would then go on to treat approximately 5,000 patients with CFS, who came from at least 48 states and 15 countries. He also published numerous articles in peer reviewed medical journals and lectured around the world on the subject of CFS. In addition, Dr. Cheney authored or co-authored publications and scientific presentations in many fields relevant to CFS, including immunology, virology, clinical epidemiology, metabolism, neuropsychology, neuroendocrinology, and exercise physiology. ~~

(2) Circa 2013, Dr. Neil Nathan was a well-known CFS and chronic illness specialist, as well as the author of several books on health and medicine. Dr. Nathan was also seeing approximately 90% of his CFS patients test positive for toxic mold toxins. After last practicing medicine in Redwood Valley, California, Dr. Nathan appears to now be semi-retired and only doing consulting work.

Note: Dr. Nathan has said he first met Dr. Brewer in the late 1980s at a lecture that Dr. Brewer was giving on his groundbreaking work showing the effectiveness of using transfer factors in treating HHV-6. It appears they became friends after that, and since then they have gone forward in sharing their medical experience and knowledge with each other. ~~

<u>Office Visit #19 with Dr. Brewer on June 24, 2014:</u>

In my notes for the doctor:

a. I tried the itraconazole for a second period, from mid-January to mid-May. The results I have seen are (1) my chest pain has still not returned, and (2) now I don't wake up in the morning feeling like I am at *Death's Door*. I may still feel *very* sick, but not *that* sick. It may not sound like it, but that's a big improvement — even if I have almost no energy at all to go with it.

b. I started the nystatin antifungal on June 18. [The nystatin was a new antifungal that Dr. Brewer was using, and he obviously believed it might serve me better than my being on the amphotericin, which we had discussed switching me over to at our last office visit.]

c. Because I believed it possible that something in my body could have been interfering with the effectiveness of my old mold medicine (the itraconazole), I started on a new anti-mold diet, of which there are two. The only difference between the two is that in one you exclude fruit. Otherwise the diet excludes wheat, gluten, high fructose corn syrup, and cane and beet sugar (and alcohol, etc.). I had been experimenting with this.

After a review of my files and my health situation, I told the doctor I was only taking the nystatin every other day because it took me a day in-between to recover from the effects of the drug. Dr. Brewer said he thought that my feeling worse, on the day after each dose, was due to a die-off reaction from the activity of the antifungal.

Dr. Brewer: "We haven't been at the nystatin very long. It just became available in early April. I've probably prescribed it for about 50 of you. But again, nobody's been on it very long. What we've heard so far is, absolutely no nasal irritation … at all, which has been a huge issue with the amphotericin.

"We have, you'd make about number four now, we've had several people that have had a die-off reaction. Now we've had a lot of people that haven't noticed anything, in terms of the die-off. We've had about three or four others who called in, and they did have the die-off reaction. So what we've told them to do is to go to every other day, [which] is exactly what you should have done. And then, if [the die-off reactions] subside, then you can move back to daily. …

"[With the amphotericin], about a third of the cases get really substantial nasal side effects — the burning, and the nose bleeds, and all of that — and had to stop it. Of the group that could stay on it, which was about two-thirds of the patients, about 90% have improved. It's very dramatic."

He went on to give a couple of patient examples.

Dr. Brewer: "The hope with the nystatin is, that it would not irritate the nose. That appears to be a slam dunk; it is not irritating the nose at all. We've heard that from everybody. And then [we hope] it will work as well as the amphotericin. Now obviously the bar's pretty high with the amphotericin, because it's 90%, but 90% of those who can stay on it.

"The other cool thing about the amphotericin is, the people who stayed on it regularly and improved, on about 20 of those we've repeated the urine levels on the mycotoxins. And they've gone down dramatically. Some of them are approaching zero, on the urine levels.

"The itraconazole does work, but I don't think it works as well as the amphotericin. Part of the reason is, it doesn't get into biofilm very well. Of course, we think a very huge piece of this is the biofilm that's in the sinuses. The mold's entrapped in the biofilm. Now of course the chelating [agent] is supposed to break up the biofilm and then allow the antifungal to get in."

The doctor went on to discuss how a few patients had fared on the itraconazole. Some of them were not better at all, but others had showed dramatic improvement. And then we talked about how I'd done on the itraconazole, with me maybe getting a little bit of a bump from it. However, I remained very sick. So, going to the nystatin was, for me, "absolutely the right way to go."

The doctor went on to discuss all the antifungal drugs he'd been using: the nystatin, the amphotericin, and the itraconazole.

Then he said: "We have to be on the right track. I mean, to have over a 100 patient's improve, come on now. Nobody's ever seen that with CFS. It's phenomenal. And I've got people that are well. I have people who are back to normal health.

"One of the big questions that comes up is, 'How long do they have to stay on this [before] they can stop it?' We've had some patients who have stopped because they felt well. And a few of them have gotten a repeat urine test, and it was real low, so they stopped. They thought, 'Well, maybe I'm cured. Maybe I don't need to take this any more. I've gotten rid of the mold problem.' They have virtually all relapsed.

"That's only at about a six month duration of therapy. … That's less than a year of therapy, probably a six to eight month time frame. So I think what we've shown is, six months is not enough. I don't know if they'll have to be on it the rest of their life, but they're going to need to be on it longer than six months.

"The other cool thing is, the people who have stopped and got worse, and went back on it, rapidly improved when they went back on it. Sometimes within one to two weeks, they felt better going back on it. So what we think is happening is, we killed down the amount of mold that was in their sinuses, but we obviously didn't get it all. It's sort of like pulling up a weed in your yard. If you don't get the roots, it grows back again. We didn't get rid of all of it, and we don't know how long it takes."

…

Bob: "In this book on mold that I'm reading, it says that the nystatin has a similar structure to the amphotericin. Is that why it should work as well as the amphotericin?" Dr. Brewer: "Yes. It kills the mold by the exact same mechanism. It works on the cell membrane. Yes, it's a similar structure. ...

"The other thing ... So let's say your die-off reactions go away, and you're not having those anymore, and you're starting to feel a little bit better. The other thing is, we're not dose-limited on the nystatin. I can give you as much as I want. It has zero systemic absorption; none of it gets in your body; it's totally safe, and there's no upper dose limitation."

Which he said was not true with the amphotericin. "I'm limited on the amphotericin, not because of systemic toxicity, but because of local side effects on severe irritation of the nose. And that's for the people who can stay on it." ...

We talked about my switching over to the nystatin recently. Dr. Brewer: "Let's face it. You're sort of like starting over again. ...

"[And, as] you get [the mold in the sinuses] killed down, there's less of it to die-off, so you don't get as much of a die-off reaction."

So after a while of being on the antifungal treatment, a patient could increase the dose of the nystatin, but that was not true with the amphotericin. Because of this, Dr. Brewer said: "I think the nystatin gives us tremendous flexibility with what we can do.

"So the thought would be with you, [on taking the nystatin], every other day for a while. If you can go to daily, that's fine. And then, if you're on daily for a while and you're doing well with that, then we could consider — down the line — going to twice a day, depending on how you're doing."

The doctor followed up by saying that they were looking at other options for killing off the biofilm.

Then I brought up the anti-mold diet I had mentioned in my office visit notes for the doctor, and I asked his opinion of it.

Dr. Brewer: "That's fine." Bob: "I thought I would experiment with it." Dr. Brewer: "I think you should. Play around with it; see if it makes a difference. If it doesn't, you tried." Bob: "I get the feeling it does make a difference." Dr. Brewer: "Yes, I'm good. Go for it."

Bob: "Oh. One question about the die-off. Do people sometimes feel like they have a fever with the die-off?" Dr. Brewer: "Yes."

I asked Dr. Brewer for his opinion on Dr. Shoemaker's protocol for treating patients for mold infection. He proceeded to discuss in detail his problems or concerns with that protocol, beginning with the way Dr. Shoemaker went about diagnosing his patients.

At some point, after hearing more than I had wanted to on the subject, I said, "You don't have to go into that much detail. I was just curious what you thought of it. I see these people — I'm on this discussion list — and I see what all these people are doing, seeing doctors that are doing Dr. Shoemaker. And I looked up some of the things they say, [and] it sounds like science fiction or something." Dr. Brewer: "You and I are in agreement." We both laughed at that. But then Dr. Brewer went on to say that Dr. Shoemaker had "some pretty decent science."

Dr. Brewer also went on to talk about Dr. Shoemaker's use of cholestyramine to bind toxins in the gut. Dr. Brewer said the problem with the cholestyramine was that it had all kinds of gut side effects and that most people couldn't tolerate it for very long.

Then the doctor switched gears. He asked: "Have you read our second paper? The one we published in December?" Bob: "No." Then the doctor told me how to find it on the Internet.

Dr. Brewer: "[It's in] the second paper that we talk about the sinuses. And what we did is, we asked ourselves the question, 'Do we think people like Robert have toxic mold, chronically, in their sinuses? And is that the source of where it's coming from?' In other words, your original exposure was someplace else [the 1993 floods in Manhattan, Kansas]. ... And some of the mold spores were toxic mold spores — when you were breathing in those heavy amounts of spores — [and] some of them got stuck in your sinuses. [And they] said, 'Gosh, this is a nice place, and I'm going to make a home here.' And they've been there ever since. And they'll be there the rest of your life unless we try and get rid of them.

"So what we asked ourselves is, could we go to the published medical literature, in the ENT sinus literature, and support that concept? Is there evidence that people have mold in their sinuses; can you have toxin-producing mold in your sinuses? And I tell people, read the paper and see what you think.

"And we also spend quite a bit of time in the paper talking about biofilm in the sinuses.

"So essentially the whole purpose of the second paper was to show [that] the literature supports what we're doing. … We're not making this up. This is published by the ENT doctors over the last 30 years." …

Bob: "You've seen a lot of improvement in people, and that's …" Dr. Brewer: "Oh, it's incredible. …

"Actually, one of my guys that started it about three weeks ago called in and said he was getting the die-off, or Herxheimer-type reaction, on it. And he said, 'Since I've been ill, I'm not sure I've ever been happier to feel worse.' His whole concept was, 'Oh, I didn't get die-off with anything in the past.' He's now getting die-off, and [there's] absolutely no way it can be a side effect, because the medicine doesn't get inside your body. … He said: 'This stuff is working.'"

<u>Office Visit #20 with Dr. Brewer on January 22, 2015:</u>

Note: In pre-visit activity, over Thanksgiving 2014, after five plus months on the intranasal nystatin, I became acutely ill (more so than usual) for several days. Then I started to notice small dark strips of something coming out of my nasal passages. These strips were dark, tar-like, and strong.   When I looked on the Internet, I saw that mold is normally dark and tarry.

When I called Dr. Brewer's office about this nasal discharge, his nurse told me that what I was experiencing was completely normal. That is, normal to have dying mold being passed out of the body through the nasal passages. Dr. Brewer's nurse said that 40 to 50 other patients had had a similar experience. She said this was a good indication that the anti-mold medicine was working.

By the time of this office visit, I had been off the nystatin since my Thanksgiving experience. ~~
In my notes for the doctor: I began by recounting the Thanksgiving episode I'd had with the dead mold coming out of my nostrils. However, I was sure the phone call from this past Thanksgiving and its contents had been recorded in my medical file.

Other items I listed were:
a. I feel less sick than I have been in years.
b. My fatigue remains severe.
c. I remain bedridden much of the time — due to my fatigue.
d. My chest pains have returned, and too much exertion will initiate or worsen these chest pains.

Dr. Brewer and I started off by discussing my being on the nasal antifungal nystatin from June until Thanksgiving of last year. I'd been taking one dose of the drug every third day, which was all I could stand, probably due to a die-off reaction in-between doses. I was on the biofilm-busting agent as well during that time.

We then discussed my current symptoms. I wondered if the nystatin use wasn't causing my returning chest pain. The doctor said that the drug couldn't be a problem because the nystatin wasn't absorbed by the body. If there was a problem in that area, then it was from the mold die-off.

Because I wasn't feeling much better, I wondered if I still had live mold left in my sinuses. Dr. Brewer: "If you recall our amphotericin experience … Now of course our nystatin experience is growing, and we're learning as we go along, and you're one of several that we've had on the nystatin. So I have about six or seven months experience with the nystatin, and I've got 18 to 20 months experience with the amphotericin, so we know a lot more about that. But I think you can extrapolate. They're both antifungals, and they both kill mold, and they both seem to work in the sinuses. … [But] the amphotericin [has] a lot more nasal side effects than we see with the nystatin.

"But still, until you actually go through it with patients and see what happens with the nystatin, there's still some question marks. But with the amphotericin, what we saw was, if it didn't burn their nose, it was very effective in helping the patients' symptoms. We would often see the mold toxin levels drop in the urine.

"And then, you may or may not not recall this … but when we analyzed that group of patients that were on the nasal amphotericin for a year, there were six patients in there that stopped it [after about six months] because they thought they were cured. So they thought they were done with it; they were feeling good; their fatigue and all that was gone, and they were feeling a lot better, and they stopped it. And five of the six relapsed. Went downhill again.

"So the only conclusion we can make at this point from that is, six months isn't long enough, seemingly, for most patients. How long do they need to stay on it? We don't know. So it gets back to what you were saying about your case: do we know if the mold is gone? We can't know for sure; but at least, based on what we've seen with other patients, it's pretty hard to get rid of. It's not that we can't get rid of it, but it's pretty hard to get rid of. [And hard to] get rid of quickly … meaning within a few months. And it probably takes considerably longer than that. …

"Although in general, you feel better than before you took the nystatin, my guess is that we have not gotten all of it.

"The other issue with you in particular is, the fatigue that you have, [is it] all due to CFS, which I would then say *mold?* Or are there other components?" …

He gave one example that was non-mold related.

Dr. Brewer: "Is the fatigue multifactorial; are there several things involved with the fatigue, and we're just treating one of them with the mold medication. … Or is 95% of the fatigue due to CFS, which I think is due to mold? The reason I say that is because we have people whose fatigue has gone away 100% on the nasal therapy. I've seen three people this week who are back to normal, two amphotericin and one nystatin. I mean, they exercise every day; they don't have any fatigue; they feel normal.

"Now of course, with those patients, then we get into the discussion, 'Well, how much longer do we leave them on it?' Like one patient who was in this week and feels completely normal, and the amphotericin doesn't bother them, [and] they don't want to quit. They don't want to risk going backwards. You know, the stuff's quite safe.

"The other issue is, something certainly happened, nasally, in November. You got this junk coming out of your nose, which could have been mold. I think you're probably right [on that]. But you had this gunk coming out of your nose for two weeks, even after you stopped it. I don't quite know why the dam broke. … I don't quite understand that. …

"So I think the nasal effects, obviously something kind of happened there. … But I don't think any of that is a direct side effect of the nystatin. Why do I say that? It doesn't get into your body. It goes up into your nose and comes back out. None of it is absorbed. … So it's almost impossible it's a side effect of the nystatin itself.

"However, that doesn't rule out a die-off. Die-off's a whole different ball game. Die-off with this whole thing, whether it's amphotericin or nystatin, is almost more of an art than a science. We think the die-off is very real. I think it was what was happening with you. I don't quite understand why you had this kind of weird sequence of events in November, but I do think that the whole pattern with you is probably that of a die-off.

"We have seen some people on nystatin where the die-off just persists. I'm not saying it's going to go on for two or three years, but it does go on for months. So you're not the only one. [Even at taking only one antifungal dose] every third day, you'd still get a die-off."

The doctor then told me the time between doing the chelation and doing the nystatin doses, which had been set at five hours between the two doses, could now be shortened to as little as 30 minutes to an hour. And this shortened time period between the two doses had not been reported to be a problem with patients who had made this change.

The doctor then discussed a patient who had also been on the nystatin. He said her die-off experience had been getting shorter in length — in-between her doses of once every three days — the longer she had been on it.

Dr. Brewer: "My suggestion [to you] would be to try [the nystatin] again, [and] try it only on every third day again. ...

"The other thing is, Robert, the number one symptom to [improve], in the patients who get better, is fatigue. Now obviously I've seen everything get better. I've seen headaches get better; pain get better; cognitive get better; twitches and muscle spasms get better. I've seen all the symptoms get better. But the single most common symptom to get better is fatigue. Which has not happened in you, and you're not feeling well."

We then discussed some alternative mold therapies I'd heard about, which Dr. Brewer wasn't very impressed with.

Dr. Brewer: "I think 95% of your problem is die-off. The thing is, you feel better. Your fatigue is still bad, and you're still getting those [inaudible] chest pains. But you're better; you don't feel like you're dying anymore. And I agree with you totally, I think the nystatin was effective. But I don't think you're rid of [the mold].

"Now if you want to do a urine test, we can do one. The repeats are $199 instead of the $500, so they are cheaper. And I'll be happy to give you a kit today, and we can do a repeat urine test. I'd love to have it, but it's your $199, not mine."

The doctor did give me a test kit to take home with me. Even if I didn't do the testing right away, I'd still have the test kit on hand for later use.

Dr. Brewer: "I think we're on the right track with you and several hundred other people. ... We're continuing to be pretty excited about this. I mean, the dots are connecting, and a variety of the treatments we're trying are working, and there's tweaking. Like [we're learning] with you, we've got to be careful with the die-off reaction." ...

<u>Follow up to my January 2015 Office Visit:</u>

In early February, I got my second RealTime Labs *Mycotoxin Panel* test results back that Dr. Brewer had ordered for me. (The testing for the gliotoxin mycotoxin was still about a year away at this point.)

The test showed that the two mycotoxins that I had tested positive for earlier — the ochratoxin and the trichothecene — were each approximately three times higher than on my initial June 2013 RealTime Labs test. I wondered how this could be, after I had passed so much dead mold out of my nasal passages. So I wrote Dr. Brewer a letter asking him about this.

Dr. Brewer said, in his response dated March 3, 2015: "Firstly, there is a lot of this that we do not know for sure. We have seen patients that stop the intranasal therapy and had the mycotoxins go up higher than the original levels. Remember that these are the mycotoxins that are coming out the body in the urine. There are many factors that can increase the output of the mycotoxins from the body (including the sauna therapy that we had discussed). [We hadn't discussed any sauna therapy at that point, but we would at our next office visit.] In your particular situation, this could represent that you are flushing out more of the mycotoxins. There could also be an element of 'regrowth' of the mold in the sinuses. There may even be a 'rebound effect' with the mycotoxins going up after the treatment.

"At no time have we ever found a strict correlation between the severity of the patient's symptoms and the actual mycotoxin levels. Again, remember these are the amount of mycotoxins that are coming out of the body. We are not doing blood levels here; we are measuring urinary excretion. Whatever the case, there is not an exact correlation with the elevation of the levels and the severity of the patient's illness. I have some patients who are extremely ill (bedridden) and have very low levels of mycotoxins. I have some patients that feel pretty good and go to work every day and have extremely high mycotoxin levels. Therefore, I think you are putting way too much emphasis on the 'percent rise' of the mycotoxin levels. I have no concern about the validity of Real-Time Laboratories, and I think their test is absolutely accurate and valid. What is not particularly clear is our understanding of the dynamics of these mycotoxins as they move in and out of tissues, into the bloodstream and out through the urine. Furthermore, we do not understand the dynamics of how they get absorbed through the sinuses with and without intranasal antifungal therapy.

"Certainly there is a lot we do not fully understand. The most important thing is that the mycotoxins are still present. The levels are probably not that important. Obviously, in all the patients we would eventually like to get the mycotoxins down to zero. That may take a considerable amount of time and emphasis on both eradicating the mold out of the sinuses as well as mobilizing all the mycotoxins out of the tissues, such as what we are trying to do with sauna therapy."

<u>Office Visit #21 with Dr. Brewer on July 28, 2015:</u>

In my notes for the doctor:

a. In January, a dental MRI of my jaw area showed my sinus cavities were clear except for one unidentified circular spot. Ten days later, I passed a sizable and translucent *thing* out of my nose. It was closed and circular at one end; but the rest of it had four walls, like legs; and it appeared the bottom of it had been blown out, or it was simply missing. I thought this might be the *biofilm covering* that had been protecting the mold in my sinus cavity. [This was contrary to what Dr. Brewer had previously said to me about the biofilm, which was that it was "kind of a gel-like substance." Perhaps that was why Dr. Brewer didn't comment on this during my visit.]

b. I got a new mycotoxin test done, and I saw I was detoxing mycotoxins at a rate three times higher than on my original test. After getting Dr. Brewer's letter on this, I began to believe that the mold was dead and I was simply having a lot of mycotoxin detox from mycotoxins absorbed some time over the 22 years I'd been sick.

c. During this time, up until the end of March, while I didn't feel very sick, I remained bedridden much of the time — with severe fatigue and daily chest pain.

d. During April, my severe fatigue gradually lessened, until I felt like I was more tired than fatigued; and my daily chest pain tapered off to occasional episodes. So I remain fatigued, with a lot of trouble in getting to sleep.

After a review of my file and my office visit notes, I asked: "If the mold is actually killed off, does your body then release the mycotoxins that are in your tissues?"

Dr. Brewer: "I think this is actually how it works. ... It's what I call the input/output model of the mold toxins. ... On the internal input, the question is — which is a bit up in the air with all of you — after a course, however long that course is, of nasal antifungals, did we get rid of all of it? In other words, did we clear the mold itself out of the sinuses?

"Now the output side is getting the mycotoxins, the poisonous chemicals that are in the tissues, getting them out of your body. ... Now obviously your body detoxes and does that naturally. That's why we get a positive urine test. So that is an ongoing, daily cleansing function that your body does. ...

"See, if there's no new input, or minimal new input from the environment and your sinuses, and your body keeps cleansing, then obviously, over time, you should get rid of most or all of [the mycotoxins]. And it was intriguing, that when we checked you in February, there was a lot coming out. Those were very high levels coming out. Which is good that they're coming out. Obviously, at some point in time, you'd like to see those levels near zero, and staying near zero."

"So one of the things that we're looking at is to enhance detoxing, cleansing, the movement of the toxins out of the body, particularly out of the tissues."

The doctor continued by saying that, when the toxins are floating around inside your body, it's highly likely they get absorbed into your tissues — with those tissues being mainly muscles and fat.

"It means they're out of the blood stream and into the tissues. And again, some of those are moving out every day, because that's when we get a positive urine test. So then the question is, can we move them out faster than your body would do on a normal day-to-day basis on its own?

"The thing we've been looking at is using sauna heat. Now when we talk about sauna, basically what I'm talking about is called *far infrared sauna,* the FIR saunas, which are the dry saunas. Those are not the steam saunas. Far infrared isn't as fancy as it sounds. The infrared heat is the heat from the sun. ... It turns out that probably the more intense heat is in the far infrared wave forms, and that appears to be the best for detoxing.

...

"There's some interesting research going on with both the near infrared and the far infrared for disease states, and [it's all in its infancy]. … For detoxing, the main focus for somebody like you would be the far infrared. …

"We know that the far infrared wave forms penetrate deep down into the tissues. So what we think is happening is that deep penetration of the far infrared wave forms is freeing up and mobilizing the toxins, and then you're peeing them out at a higher level. They're getting out of your body faster. Now, if you use a sauna, then there's actually going to be a second mechanism for getting rid of the toxins, and that's sweating. …

"So myself and some other doctors have actually done some post-sauna urine levels, fairly immediate post sauna. So the patient will do a sauna; and then, within two to four hours afterward, we'll collect a urine specimen and send it to Texas. And the levels just skyrocket. They'll go up 5 to 10 times baseline.

"Of course, your February levels were pretty high anyway, so if you took those times 10, you'd have the highest ones I've ever seen. …

"You are correct in some of the stuff you're saying in your notes, in that when you're moving those toxins out of your body, you are detoxing. [And] it can cause the patient to feel worse. Because the toxins are mobilizing. They're going through the blood stream; they could be causing issues in the blood stream, and then they're leaving your body. So some people actually feel like they're having a die-off, or a Herxheimer, or a detox reaction with the sauna. Not everybody does that.

"Now I've only been kind of heavy-hitting on the sauna since February. So like yourself, most of my patients I see every six months. And the ones who have started doing saunas, I haven't seen a lot of them back in follow-up. But I've seen a few. What I've heard so far has actually been quite positive. People think that it's helping. They think that they're feeling better. It's certainly a well documented way to detox." ...

The doctor went on to say you can also detox more than mold toxins when you do a sauna, such as detoxing heavy metals and other toxic substances that you may have gotten from the environment.

Bob: "So when this stuff comes out of your tissues and moves through your system, that can make you sick?" Dr. Brewer: "Yes. But temporarily. Usually a day or so. Sometimes just a few hours. ... Some people only feel better. ... It varies highly from one person to the next. ...

"So, for everybody, there's several different [infrared] sauna options. ... [But] what brands? How much do they cost? Where do I go get them? Etc."

The doctor said he was a rookie in this area right now, but he did go on to discuss the infrared sauna options in more detail — such as the various shapes and forms of the saunas. These included the expensive home, person-sized box; and from there it went down to the less expensive, what he called *soft-sided* or *non-firm* structured saunas. From the latter there were three options: sauna mats, sauna tents, and sauna blankets. Of course, your head and neck don't go inside any of these soft-sided sauna models.

The doctor went on to mention a local place where you could buy whatever sauna you'd like to use. That place was planning on offering discounts in pricing to Dr. Brewer's patients; and "No," Dr. Brewer would not be receiving kickbacks from any such sales to his patients.

"So the sauna thing has really turned out to be quite interesting. It seems like, if we just follow your story line that you typed out today, you have been doing detoxing on your own. I mean, you are slowly getting better; you still have fatigue and so forth, but you're making headway. And we might be able to speed that up with the sauna. So you may be at a point were you don't need to do the nasal stuff anymore. Because, the point is, can you just finish this up on your own? You can. We proved in February you're peeing this stuff out like crazy.

"So if you're still putting [all these toxins] out at a regular basis, you are and will detox on your own. But how long is that going to take? Is this going to be 10 more years? Think about it. If you put this stuff out 10 times as fast, that shortens the detox interval by a lot. I mean, you're talking about one tenth the amount of time."

I told the doctor I might be interested in this therapy, and he thought it could prove to be helpful. He went on to describe the sauna mat he thought would be good for me. However, he said he still needed to get more information from the company to know more himself.

On the FIR sauna therapy, Dr. Brewer said: "You're going to want to start out slow. We tell everybody, no matter what kind of sauna they get, we tell them to start out only about 10 minutes twice a week. Something like that. Start very slow. Because you don't know how your body's going to detox. Your body may say, 'Oh, boy, that's too many toxins at once.' ... You can obviously pick up the pace quickly if it doesn't bother you. But if there's kind of a detox reaction, then people want to go slow and let their body adapt to it.

"Maximum, really being aggressive with it, would probably be 30 minutes, five to seven days a week. ... You will want to shower off afterwards, because you want to get that sweat off your skin."

The doctor then moved on to a new but connected topic. "So one other thing I just started looking at, I think mold is what starts all of this. But how everything connects is still interesting. So this ... has to do with maybe trying another supplement.

"So over your years of reading about CFS, have you every found any of the work by Dr. Simpson? In New Zealand? About the shape of the red blood cells?" Bob: "Yes." ...

Dr. Brewer: "Some of this stuff about sauna has to do with blood flow too. Because you're getting blood flow through your tissues. If you heat yourself up, you're going to get increased blood flow through your tissues, and your muscles, and so forth.

"So that's probably how I kind of got started into it. … So in the last month or so, I've basically read all of his stuff. … What he basically showed was the vast majority of [patients with] what he calls ME — Myalgic Encephalomyelitis, but what we call in this country CFS — the vast majority of them have these funny shapes of their red blood cells. Now what that does is, it makes those cells stiffer.

"So the average, smallest of your capillaries, which take the blood way deep into your tissues, is about 4 microns in diameter. The average size of a red blood cell is 8 microns in diameter. Well, that red cell isn't going to fit through there unless it's flexible and pliable and can deform. So it turns out that flexibility, in what they call *deformability*, is a normal phenomenon for red cells. So normal healthy red cells will fit through a smaller space. They're flexible and they deform. So they'll change their shape. They will kind of go from round to oblong to slide through there. …

"What Simpson believed — and he had good data to back it up, an extensive number of papers published — is that a lot of the problems with CFS are problems with the microcirculation, meaning the capillaries. And you don't get enough oxygen to your tissues through the capillaries. It's kind of like that thick blood thing I measured you for [back in 2006]; and I think that's part of it, but it turns out there's more to it than [that] … because

I was talking about blood getting so thick it might clot. I do think that's a factor.

"But now, if you go back and look at Simpson's work, it's more complicated than that. Because he's talking about, the red cells won't fit through the small pipes, if you will. You're not getting oxygen into the tissues. And then, of course, the mitochondria are going to start malfunctioning because they're not getting oxygen. So a lot of this fits with a lot of the data that's been published about tissue oxygenation, mitochondria, and so forth.

"So what Simpson was looking for … Again, he looked at thousands of blood smears over the course of 20 years. In thousands of ME patients, he looked at their blood smears and found that consistently you could find their red cells had a funny shape.

"Now this is interesting too. He also found, like we've all reported over the years, many CFS people will kind of go up and down; they'll wax and wane; they'll have good days and bad days. He also found that, on a good day, their red cells looked more normal; and on a bad day, they were really misshapen.

"So he looked at ways to get the red blood cells more flexible. And late in his career, looking at all this, his main thing he proposed was evening primrose oil. He found evening primrose oil would restore some, if not all, the flexibility of the red cells, seemingly in about 70% of the cases.

"So you're one of the first two or three people I've told about this. A lot of people have read about Simpson over the years, but they haven't done a lot about it. I think, actually, in Australia and New Zealand, a lot of people tried evening primrose oil.

"Now Simpson also said — again I'm paraphrasing, or kind of quoting what he said — he said, first of all, some of the brands are not very potent, and some of the brands are not as good as others.

"Of course, he was doing most of his work in New Zealand, so these were brands that people have obtained in New Zealand. But some of that could apply here. So one is the potency of it; and number two, he said you have to take enough. He was talking about taking 4,000 mg a day. That's a lot.

"So the other thing that I've looked at … There are some oil supplements now that contain a mixture of oils, including sunflower seed oil, safflower oil, evening primrose oil, etc. One that I actually take myself is YES Oil, because it's supposed to be very healthy for your cells and so forth. There's a whole bunch of research behind that. But it basically would probably do the same thing.

"So the question is, should you take an oil mixture that has both the omega-3s and the omega-6s in there — of which evening primrose is an omega-6 — or should you just take the pure evening primrose? I don't know. Some of my patients will probably try taking the evening primrose, and some of them may just take the other oil. We'll see.

"This is different. This is very important now. This is different than taking fish oil. Fish oil is pure omega-3s, and evening primrose is an omega-6, so it's very different. Fish oil will not do this.

"So this is interesting too. Late in his work there was another group, I believe from New Zealand, that actually found out what's probably wrong with the red cells. Basically what they showed was, the red cells are under oxidative stress. You know, the whole thing with CFS has been that you're under oxidative stress, with too much super oxide and so forth being produced; and that's essentially kind of the same as inflammation. So the inflammation and the oxidative stress is probably damaging the red cell membranes, or at least making them out of whack. And that's been very well established.

"So the current thinking is that Simpson was right. The red cells have a funny shape, and they don't fit through capillaries very well. That leads to poor oxygen to the tissues. And the reason the cells aren't flexible enough is because they've been damaged by oxidative stress. So then the question is, what creates the oxidative stress? In my opinion, it's the mold toxins. And we have extensive data that mold toxins create oxidative stress. I could show you a 100 papers on that. That's not even debatable."

Bob: "That's caused by the mycotoxins?" Dr. Brewer: "The mycotoxins, yes, we think cause the oxidative stress. So I think it might be another [of the] dots that are linking together. Now again, if you could clean out all the mold toxins, the mycotoxins, your red cells would probably go back to normal and you wouldn't have to worry about it.

"So it could be, if we just get rid of the mold toxins, we get to the same spot. We get to the same end result. The patient feels better; they have better circulation; their mitochondria work better, and the patient overall is going to do better.

"The only reason I'm telling you is, I think Simpson was right. And if you took a supplement like evening primrose oil, or one of the omega-6 containing oils, and it would make you feel better, that's good. That gets you to where you want to go faster.
…

"You know, you're getting a little bit better as each few months go by.

"Back to this oxygen stuff. Boy, would that explain your shortness of air and stuff. Because you're getting signals going to your brain and saying, 'We're not getting enough oxygen.'"

Bob: "I think I read a study somewhere that said the capillaries, because you're not getting enough oxygen to the brain, causes brain fog." Dr. Brewer: "Yes. That causes the brain fog. And the other issue is, people like you almost always have abnormal SPECT scans, and SPECT scans are blood flow. So Simpson actually wrote that in his work. He thinks the abnormal SPECT scans are due to the poor blood flow in the brain, which symptom-wise causes brain fog, and on imaging causes an abnormal SPECT scan.

"The big question is, what set's all this off? What deforms the red cells? What causes the oxidative stress to their outer membranes and so forth? And I think, from the data we're collecting, probably the mold toxins."

Dr. Brewer then recounted two more cases where his patients had fully recovered their health: one who did only the nasal antifungal, and one who did both the nasal antifungal and the sauna.

Bob: "So are we looking at, if I try the sauna, as long as I don't start going back downhill, then I don't have to worry about taking the mold medicine?" Dr. Brewer: "Yes. [But] remember, if you go downhill temporarily, after the sauna, that's detox. You understand that, right?" Bob: "Yes." Dr. Brewer: "[Then] that's correct. We would hold off [on restarting the antifungal nasal treatment]."

Bob: "Should I take a test kit with me just in case?" Dr. Brewer: "Yes. … Let's not do it right away, but we might want to do it before next time. You'll have the kit at home. Those kits last forever, so that's a good idea."

As far as getting some sort of sauna, if I was interested, I was to call Dr. Brewer after another week had passed. He expected to have more information on them by then.

In closing, I asked, "If I do the evening primrose oil, how high a dose could I go?" Dr. Brewer: "You can go up to 4,000 mg."

<u>The Two Newer Published Papers by Dr. Brewer et al:</u>

(1) <u>https://globaljournals.org/GJMR_Volume15/5-Intranasal-Antifungal-Therapy.pdf</u>. "Intranasal Antifungal Therapy in Patients with Chronic Illness Associated with Mold and Mycotoxins: An Observational Analysis," by Joseph H. Brewer, Dennis Hooper & Shalini Muralidhar, University of St. Lukes Hospital, Kansas City, Missouri, United States. Published in: Global Journal of Medical Research: K Interdisciplinary Volume 15 Issue 1 Version 1.0 Year 2015 Type: Double Blind Peer Reviewed International Research Journal Publisher: Global Journals Inc. (USA)

(2) <u>https://globaljournals.org/GJMR_Volume15/6-Intranasal-Nystatin-Therapy.pdf</u>. "Intranasal Nystatin Therapy in Patients with Chronic Illness Associated with Mold and Mycotoxins" by Joseph H. Brewer, Dennis Hooper & Shalini Muralidhar, University of Missouri - Kansas City, United States. Published in: Global Journal of Medical Research: K Interdisciplinary Volume 15 Issue 5 Version 1.0 Year 2015 Type: Double Blind Peer Reviewed International Research Journal Publisher: Global Journals Inc. (USA)

Note 1: The *significant improvement* numbers that I opened this book with I took from these papers. The first paper reported 94% of patients treated with the amphotericin B, and the second paper reported 83% of patients treated with the nystatin, showed clinical improvement with their respective therapies.

(In a radio interview in 2015, Dr. Brewer said that patient improvement meant that "they improved by at least a 25% reduction in their symptoms.")

These numbers only included those patients who didn't have to discontinue the intranasal therapy due to intolerable adverse side effects, with such discontinuation being experienced in a remarkably high 34% of the amphotericin B group.

Note 2: In the first of the two papers above, in the study using the nasal amphotericin B antifungal for therapy, there were 94 patients who completed the treatment, and 88 of those patients showed at least a 25% improvement in their symptoms. And out of those 88 patients, remarkably 26 (or 29.5%) of them said they had returned to full, or near full, normal health. ~~

<u>Letter from Dr. Brewer dated October 22, 2015:</u>
In response to a letter that I wrote to Dr. Brewer on detoxing, Dr. Brewer replied (in part):

"It is almost undoubtedly that you are slow to clear toxins. Recently, we have been looking at the MTHFR gene mutation since it is heavily involved with methylation, the ability to generate glutathione and detox capabilities. We have found that almost everybody with mold has the MTHFR mutation. This data is early, but we will be collecting more data over the next few months.   Obviously, with the mutation there may be some benefit from trying methyl folate and the specific forms of B12 (either methyl B-12 or Hydroxo B12).   If you want to get the laboratory test done, we could certainly have it ordered. Unfortunately, in the patients who are genetically slow to detox, there are limiting things we can do other than to take things really slowly.   That would include the nasal treatment and sauna."

Dr. Brewer appeared to be telling me that, if I had this particular gene mutation, then I couldn't properly detox the mold toxins out of my body, which was a major goal of my treatment.

So, per Dr. Brewer's letter, and using my own judgement, in early November I started taking Jarrow brand B-Right capsules, with each capsule containing 400 mcg of methyl folate and 100 mcg of methylcobalamin (methyl B-12).   I took this supplement twice a day.

In late November 2015, a local lab ran a MTHFR Mutation PCR test on me, which was fully paid for by Medicare.   On December 2, I heard back from Dr. Brewer.   He said that my MTHFR genetic analysis was abnormal, with two mutations.   He further said: "This will reduce your enzyme activity of MTHFR by about 50%. This could be very significant in your illness."

The doctor then gave me his recommendation for methyl B vitamin supplementation that he suggested I try.   It was as follows:

a. From the Seeking Health brand, Active B12 with L-5-MTHF lozenge. It has 1,000 mcg of methyl B-12 and 800 mcg of active methyl folate.

b. Start slow and work up to full doses. Start with 1/4 tablet sublingual two to three days a week, working up to 1/4 lozenge daily.

c. If (or when) that is well tolerated, gradually increase by 1/4 of a lozenge per day until you reach a full lozenge daily.

d. The reason for the slow ramp up is to avoid an excessive detox reaction.

I reported back to the doctor that up to the end of November, after 30 days on the methylation supplement, I was was feeling surprisingly better. However, by the time I had received the doctor's letter of December 2, I was feeling much worse. I sensed that I had begun detoxing much that my body wasn't able to detox before.

On December 9, I received another letter from the doctor. He said it was apparent I was on the wrong dose of the methyl B vitamins and taking them too often. I went ahead and ordered the Seeking Health brand supplement that was suggested by Dr. Brewer. With this new supplement, I would cut back on both my dosage and frequency of use.

By Christmas, my health was up and down, but I was sleeping better. And I even had one whole day where I had felt *normal.* Then, during January, I'd had either bad days all day long, or days where I was swimming in and out of feeling better and feeling worse.

Office Visit #22 with Dr. Brewer on January 19, 2016:

In my notes for the doctor: I listed my experiences on the methyl B vitamins since my last visit.

After a review of my file and my visit notes, Dr. Brewer began our visit by saying that he and Dr. Neil Nathan had talked about methylation quite a bit. That Dr. Nathan "had done a study with methylation and CFS patients, using these low doses of methyl B-12 and methyl folate and so forth."

Dr. Nathan and Rich Van Konynenburg (a PhD and CFS researcher, now deceased), "at the time they did their study back in about 2011 or so, thought that what you have listed here [in my visit notes] is correct; that it was opening up the methylation pathway and detoxing too fast. That there are stored toxins in the body, and that they're being released out of the tissues too much at a time, and it's overloading the system, and the patient is feeling worse. That was their thought.

"[Dr. Nathan] said treating these people with the methyl B-12 and the methyl folate is very frustrating because some of them are just hypersensitive to it and others are not.

"So you're one of the first ones that I've seen back. People ask me, 'How are the people doing on it?' I don't know. We've had a couple of phone calls where people felt worse, and we had to cut the dose back.

"I probably have at least 75 patients trying it. We haven't had a lot of feedback. I did hear from a guy yesterday that said that he was feeling substantially better on the vitamins. And he'd worked up to pretty much a full pill a day. So some people are just really sensitive to this stuff, even in small doses. I've read that before, and I've heard it repeatedly from Dr. Nathan. …

"So the leading thought is, what you said is correct. It is detoxing too fast, basically, to put it in simplistic terms. It's a little hard to figure out with you. … You did pretty well for about a month. But while still taking that, you started …" Bob: "I think I was taking too much." Dr. Brewer: "Right."

We then discussed the dosage of the methyl B vitamins I'd been taking.

Bob: "I think, when I get constipated, it makes me sicker. And I'm really struggling with this constipation." We went on to discuss my constipation and my using MiraLAX for it.

Dr. Brewer: "I think that might be a big deal from a couple of different standpoints. So far as we know, any toxins, including the mycotoxins, get out of your body via three pathways: urine, bowels, and sweat. And when you're constipated, that takes one out of the loop."

I brought up that I think the toxins also come out through the skin without the sweat, because of the skin rashes I got sometimes. Dr. Brewer: "There's no way to study that. … [But I do] think the constipation can be a significant role player.

"The problem with the methylation vitamins, there is no road map. It's almost like winging it. We know what to use. … You want to start slow; you don't want to open up those methylation pathways too quickly. But like I said, Dr. Nathan has indicated he's had people who can't take even a quarter of a tablet every two weeks."

We discussed what I should do next in regards to the methylation supplements. It was decided that I should go back to what I was originally taking, but maybe play around with the dose and frequency a bit.

Dr. Brewer: "For informational purposes, I've done the MTHFR blood testing on approximately a 100 patients now. … And they're like you, they're CFS patients with a positive mycotoxin assay in the urine, and about 95% have the mutation. … So I think we're on to something. This mutation appears to be very frequent in CFS/mycotoxin cases.

"Which again, that's how I got into it in the beginning. [What] makes some sense is that if you all are genetically slow to detox, one would expect there's some reason. And I tell my patients, it isn't like this is the only potential genetic contributor. There may be many different genetic factors relating to both the detox and the illness in general. But this one obviously is pretty important, since it's hitting at about 95% of my patients that are exactly like you." …

Bob: "So the thing that has struck me about this is, that I have had periods, maybe an hour or so, where I feel normal. I mean, I don't have the strength or the stamina; I can't walk very far." Dr. Brewer: "Which tells you there's reversibly in this."

Bob: "Last month, I felt so good. I cleaned my whole apartment; then I cleaned out my storage locker. It was just a wonderful day. I had energy. I felt good. But then I went back [down again]." Dr. Brewer: "Yes, it's frustrating for us too.

"But the hugely encouraging part about it is, there's no permanent damage inside of you." Then he listed the health issues I had outside of CFS. "But still, in terms of just feeling sick, flu-like sick, to have a day like that tells you that's not permanent. … The frustrating part is, it's so up and down, it's maddening. … But I think we're in kind of a positive direction."

Bob: "Well, I'm certainly having less chest pain. I have nights where I sleep very deeply. So, even though I'm sort of in-and-out of this, this feeling good an hour here and there is amazing."

Dr. Brewer: "You're not doing any nasal therapy presently, right?" Bob: "No."

Dr. Brewer: "Now the other thing I've been looking into … This is just as complicated as methylation. The approach might be a little easier, and this very interestingly might tie in with your constipation as a complicating factor. I got a fascinating paper. You can find it on the Internet. I think it's free.

"About three or four weeks ago, somebody sent me an interesting paper, just published in December, and this has to do with changes in what we call the gut microbiome in CFS patients versus the controls. Now that's actually been studied before. So the gut microbiome are basically the healthy bacteria in the gut. So this ties in with the balance of bacteria in the gut, and then gut inflammation; leaky gut; what they call the gut-brain axis, where the gut can affect how the brain functions, and all kinds of things."

Bob: "It affects your immune system, right?" Dr. Brewer: "Same thing. The immune system, etc. But it's more than that. It has to do with neurotransmitters in the brain, chemicals that are produced. … It's one of the hottest things in all of medicine right now, is this whole gut thing.

"[So, in this study,] they took 10 healthy controls and 10 CFS patients. They measured, or they looked at, the different balance of bacteria in their stools. And they also measured if any bacteria got into the blood stream, which would be what we call [gut] translocation or leaky gut, where bacteria are actually crossing into the blood stream. And then they had them walk on a treadmill. They exercised them, and they looked at what happened with the stool and the bloodstream after exercise.

"There was a difference between the two groups, pre- and post- exercise. But it was even more dramatic post-exercise. There was a difference in the stool balance, and there was a difference in what got into the blood stream. Post-exercise.

"So their thought was, maybe with exertion, CFS people are having even more marked change in the balance in the normal flora in their gut. And also, more stuff leaks across into the blood stream, and it can cause an inflammatory reaction and that sort of thing.

"So that study was interesting enough. But it got me to looking at it, and there's actually a lot published on this. I was surprised. And it kind of ties in with the fact that a high percentage of people with CFS also have irritable bowel syndrome. [And] a lot of them have bowel symptoms [that] haven't been diagnosed [as] irritable bowel syndrome. And then there's a number of studies on gut inflammation and leaky gut, and so forth, in CFS, etc. So I've been looking at that. And so I think your constipation, in some ways, may tie in with that as well, being not only a symptom, but also it makes the whole situation worse.

"Now one thing that's kind of interesting is, if you look at the mold toxin literature, the mycotoxins are very damaging to the intestinal lining. Is it possible that's the actual initial trigger that sets the gut off? That's a hypothesis, or theory, but it's an interesting thought. So let's say that it is mycotoxins. Then we're back to the whole same story again. You've got to get rid of the mycotoxins.

"But is there anything you can do to sort of change that dynamic with the gut? In other words, can you heal the gut? Can you get normal flora back in better balance? Can you make it less leaky, which would then cut down on the inflammation that's coming out of the gut; and that would then cut down on the bad substances that are getting up into the brain and so forth? There are some things, like amino acids, like glutamine and probiotics, and so on and so forth. There are some interesting ways to do it.

"Now what I've been working on for about the last week are probiotics, and I've actually learned a lot about probiotics. The problem that's confusing for me and everybody else is, there's hundreds and hundreds of probiotics on the market. It's much worse than these methyl B-12s. … Different brands and so forth.

"And since there's at least 500 species of bacteria that are in the GI tract — there's not that many species in probiotics — but there's probably at least 50 or so different species of bacteria and stuff that you could add to a probiotic mixture.

"So some of them only have one thing in them; some of them have 15 or 20 bacteria in them; they're supposed to be healthy bacteria. So which ones are the best ones? … People ask me about taking a probiotic, and I say, 'Sure, that's fine, I think it might help.' And then they say, 'Dr. Brewer, which one?' And I say, 'Just go find a good one.' …

"I'm telling you, to look into this, it takes hours and hours of work. I mean, you just have to pour over these papers, and there's a huge amount written on it. And it gets into depression, and irritable bowel syndrome, and Crohn's Disease, and ulcerative colitis.

"But I'm getting closer all the time to kind of getting a sense of which probiotics I like. So I think probably within a month I can give you a recommendation for a probiotic. So I'm trying to come up with kind of a simple little supplement formula that would have three or four things in it, one of which would be a probiotic, that would help the gut."

I told the doctor I was already taking a probiotic, but that I'd only been on it for about six weeks so far. I also told the doctor about my seeing Dr. Scott Rigden in Tempe, Arizona, after I lost my job 20 years ago. He was treating CFS patients for gut and liver problems, and he had a treatment for both of them. I didn't need the gut one, but I did need the liver one. He used a powdered supplement called UltraClear for the liver (and UltraClear Sustain for the gut). He also put me on a very strict diet, which was basically fresh fruits and vegetables, and fish. And I had felt a whole lot better after that.

Dr. Brewer: "When you change your diet to things that have a lot of fiber in them, like fruits and vegetables … the gut bacteria are always interacting with the foods that we eat. So dietary changes can be a big part of it.

"You know, there's been quite a bit of work on gut bacteria and obesity. … There's some fascinating work in mice where you can actually do a fecal transplant in a mouse and put a different balance of bacteria in their gut, and the mouse will get fat. You start out with mice that are all normal, and if you change their gut bacteria, one group will get fat and the other group will get skinny."

Bob: "Toxicity will sure put weight on you." Dr. Brewer: "Yes. For sure, for sure. So keep taking the probiotic. … [Do] you remember how many strains are in there?" Bob: "There's a bunch, like about 18." Dr. Brewer: "So that's good. Because the more you have in there, the better the chance is that we'll have some of the good ones in there. All of them are good, but some of them are better than others."

Bob: "One thing I did read is that you should buy it at a store where [the probiotic is kept] cold, and keep it refrigerated [at home]." Dr. Brewer: "Right. I've read that too, although I think there are some that are okay that are not refrigerated."

Office Visit #23 with Dr. Brewer on July 19, 2016:

In my notes for the doctor:

(1) My experience with my methyl B vitamins:

a. Since my last visit in January on through to April, I tried to find a dose of the methyl B vitamins that would work for me. By mid-April, I was taking 500 mcg of methyl B-12 and 400 mcg of methyl folate every five days. With each day, there were lots of ups-and-downs.

b. What I was seeing from those doses was that, after a couple of hours after taking a dose, I started feeling worse. Then I was usually down health-wise all the next day, and this was followed by about three days of being on a rollercoaster of health ups and downs. On the fifth day, I usually woke up and felt halfway decent. Then in the afternoon, I started my next dose of the methyl B vitamins. Two hours later, the cycle repeated itself.

c. May 1: I felt that the detox from the methyl Bs was playing havoc with my immune system. I had bronchitis that took three weeks to resolve; and concurrently, I had fungal and bacterial skin infections as well.

d. In early May: I went to a half dose of the methyl Bs every six days. After an initial three days of feeling worse, I began to feel halfway normal; my strength was good; I did a lot of activity; and my strength and feeling better didn't fluctuate throughout the day. While I still had trouble getting to sleep, my sleep was deeper and longer.

e. Memorial Day [May 30]: I changed taking the half dose of the methyl Bs to [every three days]; and I didn't seem to worsen much, except for a couple of hours after my taking the methyl Bs. My extreme constipation ended as well.

(2) HHV-6 Infection:

a. June 6: I became horribly ill. I had liver pain, chest pain, and I could hardly breathe even with oxygen. Everyone said I looked pale and very sick.

b. June 23: I went to the ER with a fever; plus I had chest pains and liver pain; and an infection (a possible UTI).

c. July 8: my nurse practitioner told me I tested positive for a HHV-6 infection, and that I had a chest infection as well.

My questions for the doctor:

a. Can we treat the HHV-6 infection? Back in 2005, I was on the Immune Care 64, and you said, "You're already taking the Immune Care 64, so that may be having a positive effect on the HHV-6." It looks like the Immune Care 64 is no longer made. Has something replaced it?

b. Back in 2008, it looked like valganciclovir (Valcyte) was used to treat HHV-6, but it was expensive. Are there any

HHV-6 drugs around today that don't cost a fortune and aren't toxic?

Dr. Brewer started out by reviewing my file and my notes, as well as my recent lab work dated June 30 that came from my primary care doctor. He mentioned that in my blood work my magnesium level was "right at the bottom of the normal range." My magnesium level was 1.8 mg/dl (milligrams per deciliter) in a normal range of 1.8 to 2.4. He said that meant that part of the time I was probably below the normal range. "You know, magnesium's important for about 700 different things inside your body, including your heart." He suggested I go back on magnesium supplements to raise my magnesium level.

We then discussed how I had been doing since our last visit. We started out by discussing my infections and the medicine I took for those infections. This included an infection back in April that I had forgotten about, and for which I was treated with an antibiotic.

The doctor discussed my type of HHV-6 test that was done on me because it was not the one that he usually used, but he said it was still a valid test. Then he said: "The problem is, what does it mcan?"

"Bob: "I've had this pain in my liver for six weeks now, and the CAT scan didn't show anything but the fatty liver. " Dr. Brewer: "And the liver blood work, you had just a mild elevation on one of the enzymes. Other than that, it looked okay."

Bob: "So I thought, with my immune system, it seemed to be problematic, with three infections, four infections, in a row, in a short period of time. And with the pain in my liver; and my mind shredded, it felt like …" Dr. Brewer: "This was in June, when you were having all these infections?"

Bob: "Yes. … I would think I would have to go back on something. I know that you said in the past that HHV-6 attacks the brain; attacks the immune system; attacks the liver; and I seem to have all three of those, plus the HHV-6 test. So it would look like I have active HHV-6."

Dr. Brewer: "Yes, the test would suggest that. All we know is that you had pain in the area of your liver. But the prior CAT scan was okay. And your liver blood tests were okay. So I wouldn't necessarily link the HHV-6 to the liver. All we know is that you had pain in that area. And we don't know that's what's going on with the brain either.

"HHV-6 is like any of the herpes viruses, including EBV. It goes dormant, and then can reactivate. I do agree with you, the HHV-6 probably reactivated with your immune system being low. … The problem with the HHV-6 and the positive test and so forth is … we don't know what you would have been baseline. You may have been positive back in January. We don't know. … So are your symptoms due to HHV-6 or something else? You know, it could be just sort of floating around as a kind of benign, innocent bystander, or it could be significant.

"In terms of treating it, you kind of hit on the things we've at least tried in the past, the antivirals or transfer factor, or both. The main place that has transfer factors now is Researched Nutritionals. You can go to their website. ... Maybe before you leave today, I'll look up and see which one they have that has HHV-6 activity. ...

"The antiviral valganciclovir, Valcyte, it's still pretty expensive, even though it's generic. It went generic several years ago. We've tried regular acyclovir, like Valtrex, or valacyclovir, in some of these patients. I've actually had it work pretty well for EBV. It's not clear how well it works for HHV-6. ...

"The options would be to do nothing ... (b) you could do transfer factors, or (c) you could try the acyclovir." ...

Note: I seemed to recall that Dr. Brewer had written a paper on HHV-6 and transfer factor years ago, and I'm sure it can be found on the Internet somewhere.

However, I will note that in an office visit with Dr. Brewer in June 2006, the doctor told me about a conference he had just attended. According to the website for the Journal of Clinical Virology — at: https://www.sciencedirect.com/journal/journal-of-clinical-virology/vol/37/suppl/S1 — Dr. Brewer gave two presentations at the "5th International Conference on HHV-6 & 7, 1–3 May 2006, Barcelona, Spain." His presentations were entitled: (1) "Experimental/alternative therapeutic approaches for HHV-6 infection" by J.H. Brewer; and (2) "Coagulation disorders in patients with chronic fatigue syndrome (CFS) and HHV-6" by J.H. Brewer.   These articles are not free, but apparently you can purchase them if you wish to set up an account first to do so.

Additionally, Dr. Brewer said back then that this had been an excellent conference with an enormous amount of information shared.   He also said there was a relatively new not-for-profit foundation formed for the purposes of research and education on HHV-6.   It can be found at the website: https:// hhv-6foundation.org. The doctor said the two big focuses of the foundation were on CFS and MS.   He mentioned it because he thought there would be some information from the Barcelona conference on that web site sometime later that summer.

The foundation also has a mailing list you can join, with periodic news on HHV-6. I joined this list years ago. ~~

Dr. Brewer switched topics. He said: "On the B-12 and folate, that has been quite a ride." He went on to talk about how his patients were doing on these supplements. Using numbers that weren't clinically accurate and something of an estimate, he said he would call it a third, a third, and a third.

Dr. Brewer: "About a third of them feel better and notice improvement in their symptoms; about a third don't notice anything, and about a third feel worse. Of the ones that feel worse, it's been pretty much like you. It occurs very early on, and it occurs with small doses. Some of them have kind of taken it really slow, like a quarter or a half of a pill, once a week, or every four or five days, like you did. And they'll finally kind of adapt to it; do okay with it. Others, it's too overwhelming and they've had to stop it. I've had probably at least 20, 25 patients that have had to stop it. And I've told them to go ahead and stop it. I don't think it's worth making you feel worse."

The doctor said one of the problems in taking these methylation supplements may be because, according to Dr. Nathan, patients were detoxing too quickly. "He may be right."

Dr. Brewer believed there was another possible concern in taking these supplements. Patients had been living with this specific problem their whole lives, and their bodies had adapted to it. Then, when these new methylation supplements got introduced, the patients' bodies got overwhelmed. "It's too much."

So with the patients who did worse, he had them stop taking the supplements. For those patients who saw no difference, he let them make the choice to stop the supplements or not. And for the patients who were doing better, he had them stay on the supplements.

As for me, Dr. Brewer said: "So if you want to keep playing with it, that's fine." He said to just keep the doses really low.

Note: As to the following question that I asked the doctor, I found several references on the Internet to papers or presentations done by Konstance K. Knox, Ph.D.; Joseph H. Brewer, M.D.; and Donald R. Carrigan, Ph.D. ~~

Q. A decade ago, Dr. Brewer had said, when he — and Konstance Knox and Donald Carrigan, PhDs — had tested his CFS patients monthly during a one year period, 90% of his patients had tested positive for the HHV-6 virus at least once. In December 2013, Dr. Brewer had said 92% of his CFS patients had tested positive for toxic mold. With the two numbers being so close in percentage, did Dr. Brewer think CFS patients get the toxic mold colonization first; then the mycotoxins from that mold attacks the part of the immune system that controls the herpes viruses, allowing for HHV-6 and/or EBV to become active, or at least periodically active?

A. "Yes. See, it's not just HHV-6, because we have other people that we think have active EBV. And our patients that have had tick bites and so forth, maybe it's Lyme that's active, or Babesia, or other things. Maybe in some people it's mycoplasma. It's all the different things that have been talked about. Yes, that's exactly what we think happens. The mold toxins suppress the immune system, [and] then other things can kick up."

Bob: "Do you think now, if someone kills off their mold, you think that could change the way the HHV-6 virus works?"

Dr. Brewer: "Yes, because the immune system may correct."

Bob: "Which means it would keep the HHV-6 under control?"

Dr. Brewer: "Sure. [And this would include both HHV-6A and HHV-6B.] But they're both controlled by the immune system: just like EBV is, and chicken pox, and everything else. They're controlled by the immune system, and a very important control mechanism is the natural killer cells, and of course yours historically have been bad. ... [So] if your immune system is normal, then the [HHV-6 and EBV] would probably remain dormant, like in normal healthy people."

Bob: "How do you know when the immune system becomes normal?" Dr. Brewer: "The first question is, can you get rid of the mold and get rid of the immune suppressive effect? One of the things that we're looking at — it's a slow, methodical process — but one of the things that we are doing is to repeat the natural killer cell test. ...

"We probably ought to have this other conversation first about some of the new mold stuff, but let's say you get rid of the mold toxins. You think the mold is either controlled or gone, and the mold toxins are down to zero, or close to zero. And the patient says, 'Gosh, Doc, I feel great.' At that point then, if they've had a low natural killer cell test in the past, which most of you have had, then we'd repeat the natural killer cell test.

"There's another test we use in the Lyme patients called the CD57 count, which is a little bit like the natural killer cell test, but it's been used more with Lyme. So we do some of that immune testing to see [if we can] show on paper that the immune system is better.

"In my experience, if the natural killer cell test has been low in the past, and the patient says I still have my same CFS symptoms I've had all these years, and you repeat [the test], it's still low."

The doctor then talked about an Australian study in this area.

Dr. Brewer: "But the question is, if the culprit — which I believe to be the mold toxins — suppresses the immune system, and we get rid of the mold toxins, or get them down very low, then the natural killer cell test might correct. Now I've got a couple of them that are up in the normal range, who feel fine.

"It's so slow trying to get the whole mold thing under control that I don't have a lot of cases where the natural killers have got back to normal. And the reason I'm specifically talking about natural killers is, it's by far the most common immune abnormality in CFS. And it's one of the main control mechanisms for herpes viruses." Bob: "So if you're still detoxing mold toxins out of your tissues, that could mean that your immune system is not ..." Dr. Brewer: "Correct."

Note: The natural killer cell test Dr. Brewer refers to in our office visits is the *Natural Killer Cells, Functional* assay lab test; with the test code 34184, and which is only done by Quest Diagnostics. ~~

Q. On the website https://www.voiceamerica.com there used to be three interviews with Dr. Joseph Brewer listed, ranging in dates from 12/15/14 to 01/08/16. The interviewer was Dr. Neil Nathan (along with Dr. Jacob Teitelbaum on the first interview).

Unfortunately, I can no longer find these interviews listed on that website. Still, I have a quote that I wrote down in my notes from the encore presentation of the original interview with Dr. Brewer in 2014, which was entitled: "Special Encore Presentation: Mold Toxicity: An Important Unrecognized Cause of Fibromyalgia and Chronic Fatigue [Syndrome], New Research with Dr. Joseph Brewer." This encore presentation was dated June 5, 2015, and it was approximately 58 minutes in length.

At about 14:00 minutes into the interview, Dr. Neil Nathan said: "I am now currently treating well over 300 people with mold toxicity in their urine, and many of them are people that I have not been making progress with, with [those who have] Chronic Fatigue [Syndrome] and fibromyalgia and Lyme disease. And now, [after treating them for toxic mold infection], many of those people are making progress. As I watch their mold toxicity numbers drop, I am watching them get better."

Dr. Nathan's website is at: http://www.neilnathanmd.com.

After reading this quote to Dr. Brewer, I asked him if he had seen the same thing as Dr. Nathan in treating his CFS, fibromyalgia, and Lyme disease patients. **A.** "Yes."

Q. Has the doctor seen a decrease in pain in his fibromyalgia patients who have been successfully treated for mold toxicity?

A. "Yes. I had a patient in about three to four weeks ago. She's been on the mold treatment for about a year and a half, probably. She does the nasal, and then she did get a sauna about six months ago. Now she was doing good before she got the sauna; she thinks it's even helped her more. And she told me, and this is a quote, that 99% of her fibromyalgia pain was gone. Her brain was back to normal; she had no brain fog. And virtually all of her fatigue was gone. She wanted to make a point to me that her fibromyalgia was essentially gone. And that's not just that one case."

Dr. Brewer: "There are two new major developments on the mold and mycotoxins. One is just an FYI … and that is, Medicare now pays for the [RealTime Labs] urine test. So I'm going to give you a kit today. … Go ahead and send it in. I'll let you know about your results.

"Now that brings me to the other new development, and this is the main thing I wanted to talk to you [about] today, as it relates to the mold. As of February 1, 2016, RealTime added a fourth mycotoxin to the panel: gliotoxin. So that was added on February 1, and that's for the same price. … So all the panels we've gotten back since February, I have had four results instead of three. So we've actually gotten a lot of results back since February 1. Roughly about a 100."

Bob: "So this gliotoxin is a toxic mold?"

Dr. Brewer: "It's a toxin produced by the mold. … So there's kind of been two parallel things with regard to me and gliotoxin. Number one is, I've been tracking my results [of my patients' gliotoxin results using a spread sheet], and I'll share some of that with you in a second."

Dr. Brewer then mentioned he gave two presentations on mold in Texas back in June, and he said one of those presentations was on gliotoxins. He also said that those presentations should be up on the RealTime Labs website in the near future.

Dr. Brewer: "So what do we know about gliotoxin from the literature? Gliotoxin is made predominantly by Aspergillus. Aspergillus is one of the most common molds on earth. … It's common, both outdoors and indoors. …

"Now in terms of exposures, how people got exposed and got sick from the mold toxins, probably not very many of those were due to outdoor exposures. …

"Otherwise, probably the vast majority of exposures are indoors. … Mold testers and mold remediators will tell you the most common mold they find that produces toxins indoors is Aspergillus. Aspergillus is a very common indoor mold and can produce several different kind of toxins, including commonly gliotoxin.

"So gliotoxin's toxicity … Now listen to this closely, this is important stuff. So one definite, proven, not even up for debate, absolutely sure about, toxicity of gliotoxin is it suppresses the immune system. … And it appears to be very broadly immune suppressive. It can suppress a number of different types in the immune system: T cells, macrophages, etc. We've thought all along that all of the toxins could be immunosuppressive, but with gliotoxins, it's not even debatable. There's probably 20 papers published on that. …

"The other thing … This gets a little complicated, but we'll go through this, and I think you've done some reading on this in the past, so it'll help you out some. So this has to do with glutathione. The other thing that we think gliotoxin does is, it depletes your glutathione.

"The mechanism is, if you don't recall, glutathione is three amino acids that are hooked together. It's a little, short, tiny protein. And it's three amino acids that are hooked together: glutamine, glycine, and cysteine. The working end of the molecule is cysteine, which is an amino acid. So cysteine is where glutathione binds to free radicals, and binds to toxins, and so forth. That's the working end of the molecule.

"So it turns out that gliotoxin and glutathione interact with one another. They bind to one another. So gliotoxin will bind to, and inactivate, glutathione; and glutathione will bind to, and inactivate, gliotoxin. So it's almost this kind of vicious circle.

"But what happens is, if one has a higher level than the other … Say gliotoxin levels are too high, then that's going to eventually lead to lowering of the glutathione levels, and the patient will end up with glutathione deficiency and depletion.

"Now if you look at the literature of when glutathione levels have been measured in CFS, there are several papers showing that glutathione levels are low in CFS. Furthermore, if you look at fibromyalgia literature, same thing's been shown in fibromyalgia; as well in other disease like MS, Parkinson's, etc. They have low glutathione levels."

Bob: "Even though I've been treated for the mold, and I take this [next RealTime Labs] test, it's possible gliotoxins could show up on this test?" Dr. Brewer: "Yes." Bob: "And then I would need to treat for that?" Dr. Brewer: "Yes. And that's what's going to happen."

This caused an audible groan of discouragement from me.

Dr. Brewer: "Wait. You haven't heard my results yet. If you put gliotoxin in a test tube, and you add glutathione to the test tube, [the glutathione] will inactivate and neutralize the gliotoxin. If you do the same study, and you use NAC, n-acetyl-cysteine — which is a building block for glutathione, because it's the cysteine — it'll do the same thing." …

"So that's one of the treatments that we're doing now. We're adding either NAC or glutathione to the … we're giving them systemically." Bob: "What do you mean 'systemically?'" Dr. Brewer: "Pills. Take NAC in a pill." Bob: "So it wouldn't be a nasal thing?" Dr. Brewer: "Well, NAC is available nasally as well.

"So let's say I do a urine test on you, which we will do. And you test positive for gliotoxin, which is probably going to happen.   And we think that may be coming from Aspergillus that's colonized in your sinuses. That means that the Aspergillus is producing gliotoxin in your sinuses; it's being absorbed through the wall of the sinuses; goes throughout your body; suppresses your immune system; makes you sick; affects your mitochondria; etc. … and it comes out in your urine, and that's why we get a positive test. So wouldn't it make sense to try and inactivate it before it even gets out of the sinuses? So if we spray NAC into your sinuses, that's like a test tube. Now the NAC won't do anything to kill the Aspergillus; that's why we use the antifungals, usually the nystatin."

Bob: "Was the Aspergillus one of those three toxic molds I was tested for before?" Dr. Brewer: "We didn't test you for the mold; we tested you for the toxins produced by the mold, and the answer is 'yes.'" I was confused at this point about what I had tested positive for. I didn't think I had tested positive for any toxins that were produced by Aspergillus.

Bob: "There were three toxic molds on my test." Dr. Brewer: "Right. Aspergillus can produce two of them, and Stachybotrys produces the third one. So one of the two that Aspergillus can produce, you were positive for." (The one made by the Aspergillus that I tested positive for was the ochratoxin.)

Dr. Brewer then told me that the pharmacy he'd been using, the ASL Pharmacy, had been bought out by *Imprimis*, a national chain. He also said this pharmacy carried the nasal NAC.

Dr. Brewer: "I talked to Imprimis when I was down in Texas, at that meeting. I said, what do the ENT doctors — because they already had it on their menu; they didn't put it on there for me — what do they use it for? And they said it breaks up mucus and biofilm. So that would be another big plus.

"So the NAC, theoretically, would have two big pluses. It'll break up mucus and biofilm, and allow people to breathe better through their nose, and allow the medicine to get up in there better, the antifungal. And the new twist I've added into it is, it should inactivate gliotoxin in the sinuses.

"Now listen closely to this one too, and this again is in my presentation that'll be online. There's a test tube paper out there … published several years ago, where they took Aspergillus in a test tube, a strain that produces gliotoxin. … They put it in a test tube, and they added amphotericin to the test tube — amphotericin is one of the nasal sprays we use — and gliotoxin amounts just shoot up.

"Which, in my opinion, is exactly what we see with die-off. In other words, you're producing more toxin as the mold is dying. It's almost like that paper proves what we see with die-off. But remember what they tested for, gliotoxin? What can inactivate gliotoxin? NAC. So what we're doing now is, we're having people squirt NAC up there first, and then follow it with the antifungal. Is it possible the NAC will block the die-off? Maybe.

"See, all of this gliotoxin stuff is new. We've only been doing it since February. And the nasal NAC, I've only been doing since about June 10. Now we have not had anybody call back and say they don't like it. We've probably sent 20 prescriptions in for nasal NAC, maybe 25. So we're kind of putting everybody on the nasal NAC.

"According to Imprimis, there really isn't any down side: it doesn't have any side effects; it's perfectly safe, even if you absorb some. Then we're also putting people on oral NAC.

"Now you can use glutathione. There's a bunch of different glutathiones you can buy, like liposomal glutathione and all those. The reason I'm picking NAC is because it's easy to take; it doesn't have any side effects, and it's cheap. It doesn't cost very much. And so most of my patients do not have just an abundance of extra resources setting around. They're spending some already on supplements and meds. [So if we're going to add anything on, we want to keep it] cost effective."

"There may be some other forms of glutathione, like the liposomals and so forth, that are a little bit better than the NAC, but I'm not sure they're better enough to justify the price. I have a few people that are doing some of the other glutathiones. [But] how much glutathione, how much to take, the dosing, and how to space it out and all that? We're kind of just working on that.

"I'm starting most people out on twice a day. What we'll do with you is, once I get your results back ... I will send you a letter, with your results, which of course will have gliotoxin on there. And we'll be able to see where you're at with the other three that you had in the past. … And again, Medicare will pay for it. So once I get your results back, I'll send you a letter with your results, and I will tell you the supplements I want you to take and the doses."

We went back over the Aspergillus mold versus the gliotoxin in the urine test results. I seemed to have understood it better the second time around.

Dr. Brewer: "[Now] let me tell you what I've found so far. So I've tested about a 100 or so patients since February 1, in which we get the gliotoxin on the panel, okay? [And] 97% are positive, for just that toxin." I was stunned by the high percentage. Dr. Brewer: "Yeah, you think that's pretty stunning? That means you all have Aspergillus inside of you. Yeah, it's pretty stunning. …

"We definitely think the mycotoxins are a huge player in CFS … [and] if you sort out the mycotoxins, is gliotoxin *the* big player? Maybe. And the reason I say that is because virtually all of you test positive. …

"So the cut off for gliotoxin [to test positive] is 0.3 [ppb, or parts per billion] … and the levels I get back are high. I get 5.0, 7.0. The highest I've had is 28.0. And the cut off, remember, is point three.

"So the lady I just told you about, who said 99% of her fibromyalgia was gone, all of her toxins levels were low. The three others were below the cut off [for being positive for mold infection]; and gliotoxin was 0.5, not very high. My average gliotoxin level I'm getting back is around 4.0 ppb, parts per billion. Remember, the cut off is point three. …

"How about the lady's who's a 28? That's a 100 times the cut off. I've had a 28, a 15, a 12, a 16. I mean, I get 6s and 7s back all …" Bob: "Wow." Dr. Brewer: "I know! That's what I'm telling you. This is a big deal. This gliotoxin is a big deal. Ninety seven percent are positive, and the levels are usually high. Now a lot of those are not people on treatment.

"So let's say that we put you back on the nasal [antifungal], and we put you on the NAC and all of that. So let's say that you … start feeling some better. … So then what we can do, because again Medicare's paying for it, we can repeat the assay in say six months and see what your gliotoxin level is.

"So I've only had one repeat so far, and this lady felt crummy. [She] went on the full court press with oral NAC, nasal nystatin, etc. Which she had taken before and gone off it. And her gliotoxin was 7. And six weeks later, it was zero. And how did she feel when her gliotoxin was zero? Back to normal health." Bob: "That's impressive." Dr. Brewer: "That is impressive."

Before I left, Dr. Brewer told me the transfer factor I needed for the HHV-6 was called PlasMyc (and which is now called Transfer Factor PlasMyc — or maybe it was always called that, I don't recall). Dr. Brewer said the PlasMyc was very good against active EBV and HHV-6 infections.

The company selling the PlasMyc is at: https://www.researchednutritionals.com. Also, this company has a transfer factor for Lyme disease called Transfer Factor L-Plus.

Note 1: One definition — A transfer factor is a chemical property, taken from an animal that has already developed immunity against a certain disease, and that property is then developed into a targeted formula to support a human body's immune system against that same particular disease. (From what I understand, the animal is given the disease first, and then it develops the immunity.)

Note 2: As a patient, before you can buy any supplements from Researched Nutritionals, your doctor has to be signed up with the company. However, recently a friend of mine found another website with *some* of the Researched Nutritionals products on it. It's at: https://www.treatlyme.com/Researched-Nutritionals-Supplements-s/106.htm. ~~

<u>Mold Conference in Texas — June 3 to 5, 2016:</u>
Unfortunately, I can longer find the two presentations Dr. Brewer mentioned on the RealTime Labs website. However, my notes on the two videos are as follows:

The first talk I listened to was labeled "Treatment Approach for Chronic Mold and Mycotoxin Illness." This video of Dr.

Brewer's first presentation outlined some of the earlier research on mold and mycotoxin studies that were done before Dr. Brewer himself became interested in mold and mycotoxins. Here Dr. Brewer pointed out that CFS and the presence of mold mycotoxins had similar symptoms.

The second talk was labeled "Gliotoxin Presence in Patients." In this talk, Dr. Brewer sometimes referred back to his first presentation.

The first part of this talk was devoted to the literature/studies on the gliotoxin, including what he found in his own patients. This was very clinical/technical.

After talking about the studies, and at about 35 minutes into the presentation, Dr. Brewer talked about gliotoxin toxicity. This included things he had mentioned to me before in my office visit. It also included things that were new to me: the gliotoxins decreased the rate of protein synthesis, and were neurotoxic, and induced *elevated* apoptosis (programmed cell death).

Note: Elevated apoptosis has been identified as a symptom of CFS by one of the leading authorities on the subject, Dr. Aristo Vodjani, Ph.D., an immunologist and the CEO of the Immunocsciences Lab, Inc., Los Angeles, California. In a speech made on CFS in 1997, Dr. Vodjani said that apoptosis equaled programed cell death. In normal healthy individuals, 90% of cells are functioning and 10% are dying and recycling. However, in

CFS 50% of all the cells are dying. This is because the cellular mitochondria or cellular DNA is damaged and the cells are getting signals to commit suicide. ~~

In concluding his talk, Dr. Brewer spoke about low natural killer cells and glutathione depletion.

Note: There are two videos on the Internet of Dr. Brewer talking about CFS and toxic mold. They are entitled: (a) Dr Joseph Brewer - International Symposium on Fungal Metabolite Treatments at https://www.youtube.com/watch?v=8FNP03h2d1o; and (b) Mycotoxins and Chronic Illnesses by Joseph Brewer at https://www.youtube.com/watch?v=RxNAuk5k_Jg. ~~

<u>My History of Taking a Glutathione Supplement:</u>
I had taken notes back in 1999 on a talk given by Dr. Paul Cheney on the importance of glutathione. The talk had been given in Orlando, Florida, when I was living there. Among other things, Dr. Cheney said that glutathione was the central detoxification molecule for the cell.

The original powdered whey protein supplement — the one that was suggested by Dr. Cheney to use in raising one's glutathione levels — was a Canadian product called Immunocal. I had started taking the Immunocal back in 1999, after hearing Dr. Cheney's talk. I had noticed a boost of energy right away, on my very first day of taking the supplement.

Within days of being on the Immunocal, I felt I had recovered my health by approximately 80%.   This effect lasted for approximately six months; and then its benefits quickly faded, and I crashed back down to being very ill again.

Sometime later, I realized that, for some unknown reason, I had become allergic to the Immunocal. That being the case, it was many years before I could take it again, and by then it had been replaced by an American product called ImmunoPro. The ImmunoPro is made from cow's milk by Well Wisdom, and the company says, "It is GMO-free, hormone-treatment-free, pesticide and chemical-free and undergoes minimal processing."

I did go back on the ImmunoPro in June 2015. I started with one scoop of the supplement every three days, and later I raised it to one scoop every other day. I continued to take it well into 2018.

When I had started back on the whey protein supplement in 2015, I looked up my notes that were made circa 1999 from an Internet discussion list about how to take the Immunocal. I would think these suggestions are just as good for the newer ImmunoPro:

a. Don't take the glutathione with anything acidic (i.e., don't mix it with a Coke).

b. Don't take it within a couple of hours on either side of taking vitamin C.

c. You can mix the Immunocal with water, milk, or soy milk. Mix it with something that's at room temperature or cold. Don't mix it with anything hot, as heat destroys most of the glutathione's important properties.

d. Don't mix it with the metal blades of a blender, as the metal can cause the properties of the Immunocal to deteriorate.

e. Don't take it with food.

<u>My New Mold Test dated July 27, 2016:</u>

Dr. Brewer had me do a retest with RealTime Labs after I had seen him mid-July. He was of the belief that I needed to go back on the mold medicine, possibly because my HHV-6 flare-up indicated that my immune system was still compromised. If that was the case, it was probably due to a continuing mold infection. Of course, I'd also been very ill since June 6.

I got the mycotoxin lab test results back on August 8, 2016. This was my first test for the gliotoxin toxin, and it was *positive* for infection, coming in at 2.76 ppb. However, it was not as high as I had expected. My two other mold toxins were down from my original June 2013 mold test, with the ochratoxin down 31% and the trichothecene down 26%.

Overall, I felt that my earlier antifungal treatment had been at least partially successful, reducing my gliotoxin levels well below the 4.0 to 6.0/7.0 ppb range that Dr. Brewer had said he was seeing in most of his other CFS patients.

Robert Roy

However, with my ochratoxin, trichothecene, and gliotoxin levels still being high, it seemed to confirm Dr. Brewer's belief that I needed to be back on a nasal antifungal.

<u>Dr. Brewer Letter dated August 2, 2016:</u>
Dr. Brewer sent me a letter this date in regards to my mycotoxin lab test results. The letter said:

"The problem is what to do here. Previously, you had quite a bit of intolerance to the intranasal nystatin. At a minimum, I think we should try to get your glutathione levels up and improve that situation. That may help to some degree with the gliotoxin, and also by improving glutathione it may help move the other toxins out of your body. I would like to have you go ahead and start on oral NAC (N-acetylcysteine) 600 mg twice a day. Later on, we may move that up to three times a day. I would also like to have you add R-lipoic acid 100 mg twice a day to that regimen. These two work synergistically to recycle glutathione to its active form and raise the glutathione levels. Later on, we may want to talk about using the intranasal NAC and also give another try to the intranasal antifungal therapy such as nystatin. If we did that, we would probably need to take it pretty slowly since you had somewhat of a difficult time before. If you want to start this sooner than the next month or two, let us know, and we can always send in a prescription whenever you want us to start. I would, however, get the supplements started right away."

<u>Dr. Brewer Letter dated October 13, 2016:</u>

While Dr. Brewer believed that I needed to go back on a nasal antifungal drug at some point, I wasn't convinced. I wondered if mycotoxins detoxing out of my tissues couldn't be causing my mold-related health issues (suppressed immune system and HHV-6 reactivation) instead of mycotoxins coming from live mold still colonized in my nasal passages. So I wrote Dr. Brewer with some questions in this area, and he promptly replied. I have taken the liberty of breaking down our two letters in an effort to match his answers to my questions.

Q. How can anyone definitively tell the difference between the mycotoxins that are put out into the body from live mold colonization and the mycotoxins that are being detoxed out of the tissues? **A.** "Briefly, when the mycotoxin levels in the urine go up and down, we cannot be sure whether it is from an active mold growth (such as in the sinuses) versus mycotoxins that are retained in the tissues and are 'still detoxing' versus both."

Q. If you can't tell the difference in the mycotoxins, how does anyone definitively know where these mycotoxins are coming from, tissue detox or internal live mold? Specifically, could these mycotoxin levels last reported [on me] just be a lessening of the mycotoxins being detoxed out of my body tissues that began back in February 2015?

A. "As a general rule, as we have been through this over the last three years and looked at over 500 patients, I think that the toxin levels largely reflect new toxins coming in. The new toxins could be from the environment (such as a person living in a mold-infested environment), from the internal environment (largely the sinuses), or both.

"Again, when we find the mycotoxins coming out in the urine (no matter the level), we cannot be entirely sure of the source. We have seen patients in which the mycotoxin levels go down to very low levels (almost zero) after a prolonged course on the nasal therapy. Therefore, in your situation I suspect you may have 'internal mold' that is producing mycotoxins out of the sinuses."

Q. If I detox enough mycotoxins out of my tissues, can they do as much damage (like compromising the immune system) as a dose of mycotoxins from an internal live mold source? **A.** "The mycotoxins can do 'damage' to your immune system no matter where the source."

Note: From these answers, it seemed to me that mycotoxins being detoxed out of the tissues could be causing my health problems instead of mycotoxins coming from a live mold source. If this was the case, which I believed it to be, then taking an intranasal antifungal again would do me no good. But Dr.

Brewer disagreed, as you can see in the next question and answer. ~~

Q. Do you still believe I should be back on an antifungal drug at this point? **A.** "I do believe you should be back on an antifungal (although certainly I think intranasal is the best way to go)."

In concluding his letter, since I had tested positive for the HHV-6 a few months earlier, the doctor suggested that I "do a serology panel for EBV and see where you are on that.   It is not uncommon to have one or more of these viruses activated at the same time." I went ahead and got this lab work done.

Office Visit #24 with Dr. Brewer on January 31, 2017:

In my notes for the doctor, I summarized my experience on the valacyclovir and PlasMyc for the active HHV-6 infection. Such a summary explains why Dr. Brewer had to ask me so many questions about it during our visit. I should have provided Dr. Brewer with more detail, such as what I've done below, where I have recreated my experience with the two antivirals:

a. August 7, 2016: I started taking the Researched Nutritionals Transfer Factor PlasMyc for the HHV-6 infection at a dose of one capsule daily.

b. August 10: I started taking the NAC (N-acetylcysteine) and the oral R-lipoic acid that Dr. Brewer had wanted me on.

c. September 16: I emailed Dr. Brewer and asked him for a prescription for the antiviral drug acyclovir. Four days later I had a prescription filled for valacyclovir, and I started taking a one gram tablet daily. [It appeared to me that Dr. Brewer was using the *acyclovir* and the *valacyclovir* drug names interchangeably when he discussed my taking them. In fact, according to the Internet, they are very similar drugs. I read that the valacyclovir is converted into acyclovir in the body.]

d. October 24: I stopped taking the PlasMyc.

e. November 5: I woke up and felt pretty good; and because of this improvement, I stopped taking the valacyclovir. However, I started taking the PlasMyc again as a preventative measure.

  • In my notes for this visit, I did remind the doctor how I used to tell him that I felt sick to the core of my being, and that every cell in my body was sick and somehow they were attacking me deep inside; and also how I used to say the fatigue at times was so bad that it took great effort even to turn over in bed. But I wanted the doctor to know that on this day things had changed. I no longer felt sick to my core; I no longer felt all (or any) of my cells to be sickly. And, while I still tired easily, I no longer had such deep fatigue episodes. And, for the next 30 days, I felt like a healthy person again, but one with some lingering medical issues — instead of a person sick to the core of their being and showing medical symptoms of a deep CFS sickness.

f. November 7: Dr. Brewer notified me by letter of the results of my latest serology panel done for EBV virus. The test indicated "there could be active/reactivation EBV infection."

g. November 27: I again stopped taking the PlasMyc transfer factor.

h. December 5: I decided to *up* the doses of both my methyl B supplements (B-12 and folate) and my glutathione supplements (ImmunoPro and R-lipoic acid). I wanted to shoot for the dosages that Dr. Brewer had originally wanted me to reach. This change made me feel less well, but not overly so.

i. December 21: I got a bacterial infection and took an antibiotic for it. The effects of the infection and the antibiotic lasted through January 1, 2017, during which time I went back to being very ill.

Dr. Brewer started off by discussing with me when exactly I had been on the valacyclovir. I told him that I had started the drug on September 20 and stopped it on November 5.

Dr. Brewer: "And you took [the valacyclovir] twice a day, correct?" Bob: "I was just taking it once a day. I generally have a history of the drugs working fine for me on lower doses." … Dr. Brewer: "So you're not on it now?" Bob: "No."

As Dr. Brewer was reviewing my paperwork, I said: "It was just astonishing. I mean, November 5 to December 5, I felt so good. I didn't have a lot of strength, but I felt good. ... Then I got that infection right around Christmas, and boy I've been downhill ever since." ...

Dr. Brewer: "Now during this whole time, from August, September forward, you haven't been doing anything for the mold? ... You haven't been doing any nasal spray?" Bob: "I tried the itraconazole, and I didn't tolerate it at all." Dr. Brewer: "Nasally?" Bob: "Yes." Dr. Brewer: "What did it do?" Bob: "It just made me horribly sick, even in small doses, and even spread out over several days.

"And then we had an email exchange. And then I was going to go back on the nystatin. ... We talked about that I was probably having some HHV-6 or EBV [reactivation], or both, because I was on the transfer factor and valacyclovir, and I was probably having some die-off from that. And as soon as [the virus activity and die-off] calmed down, I was going to go back on the nystatin. But when [the virus activity and die-off] calmed down, I felt really good, so I didn't go and get a new [antifungal] prescription." ...

Dr. Brewer: "Well, I think what we should try to do is ... From December 5 until now, it's a little bit hard to know what was what because there's a lot of moving parts in there." Dr. Brewer went on to discuss the medicines I'd been on and the infection I'd had during that time. "What I would suggest we need to do is go back to exactly what you were on as of November 5. ... That month you felt really good, and you hadn't felt that way in years. What we want to try and do is recreate that."

Note: What it appears I was on at that time, before I raised my dosages on some things on December 5: 1 scoop of ImmunoPro with an R-lipoic acid supplement every three days (with my having taken no NAC after last August); one dose of 250 micrograms of methyl B-12 and 200 micrograms of methyl folate every three days (but not on the same days I took the ImmunoPro and R-lipoic acid); and generally a 1 gram valacyclovir tablet and 1 capsule of the PlasMyc daily. ~~

Dr. Brewer: "When I saw you in the summer, you had had the HHV-6 test that tested positive for HHV-6A. And then there in November, I did the EBV levels on you, and they were high and suggestive of active infection or reactivation of EBV. So, since about September, I've done a lot with EBV and HHV-6. I think more and more of these dots are connecting. So let's go back and talk briefly for a moment about the mold toxins.

"As you are aware, about a year ago RealTime Labs in Texas added on a fourth toxin to their assay called gliotoxin and started testing for that. And they added it on to their panel. So for about a year now, every result we get back has four results instead of three, the fourth being gliotoxin. The gliotoxin, in my patients with CFS and fibromyalgia and so forth, is running 99%. Virtually all of you have gliotoxin. I checked over 200 patients over the past year.

"The interesting thing about the gliotoxin is that we had talked some last time about how it depletes glutathione and that sort of thing. The other big thing with gliotoxin is that it suppresses the immune system. And it may be the most immune suppressive of all the mycotoxins. And that one's not debatable. That's not controversial. There's a substantial amount of published literature and papers on gliotoxins suppressing the immune system.

"That, of course, is not a surprise with all of you folks because we've known for years that your immune system isn't right. And that's been thought to be some of the basis of CFS. But it may be that we've actually now found the cause of the immune suppression; that it's the mycotoxins, and that they've been there all along.

"So I'm now getting stories, as I'm fishing into these stories much deeper ... that what's going on is, the mold exposure is what started all this. The mold exposure came first, for you many years ago; and that pulled your immune system down, and then something inside of your body activated. Now it could be you came across that something, and I'll use HHV-6 and EBV as examples, you could have come across that something for the first time. ... Or it could have been that the person could have picked up mono [infectious mononucleosis] when they were 12 years old; and the virus went dormant and stayed dormant, as long as they had a healthy, robust immune system. Then, when they got exposed to the mold later on, then [the virus] reactivated from dormancy.

"So what we've been doing with virtually all of my patients, since about September, is checking them for EBV and HHV-6, and we do find some patients that look like they have active HHV-6. So there is some of that mixed in there. It still could be an issue with you. Although, as I'll tell you in a moment, I think you may be predominantly EBV, given what you've just told me today. But we find a lot of people that look like they have active EBV. I mean a lot.

"So at the present time, I probably have over a 100 patients on valacyclovir. You were one of the earlier ones that I put on it because we had the viral testing that you had done last summer. But we've got a lot of people on valacyclovir now, and I haven't seen very many of you back in follow-up. You're one of probably the first five or so I've seen, so I can't share with you a lot of results. I do like what I read, though, today. I like a whole lot what I saw, November 5 to December 5. It's very positive."

Bob: "It was like a miracle." Dr. Brewer: "I think it's the antivirals, I really do. And see, the lab tests back it up. The lab tests tell us that those viruses were active when you took an antiviral.

"Now the thing is, valacyclovir, the one you took, the Valtrex, probably has minimal, if hardly any, activity for HHV-6. But it's quite good for EBV. So what I've been doing with my patients is — and insurance and so forth becomes a big problem, if we think both viruses are active — our preference would be to put them on valganciclovir, the Valcyte.   It's very expensive, a lot more expensive than the other one, and most insurances won't cover it. And then it also has more side effects. It can lower your white count and so forth.   So we have to check blood counts periodically and so forth. Whereas valacyclovir, the one that you took, it's very safe. It has almost no side effects. It's very, very safe. …

"But then we run into cases like yours, if there's evidence that both viruses are active, which one is predominating? Is it the EBV, the HHV-6, or both of them? And in your particular case, because you seemingly responded to valacyclovir, it would suggest that actually the big player is EBV.

"I don't want to get too crazy here. Let's just go back to what we were doing before.

"Now one thing I need to ask you, remind me again, which transfer factor you take?" Bob: "PlasMyc." Dr. Brewer: "And when did you start it?   I mean, have you been on it quite a while?" Bob: "I was on it before November 5; then I started it again like the 1st of January."   Dr. Brewer: "But here's my question, how long before November 5? Was it just a couple of months, or was it like six months to a year?" Bob: "I ordered it at the same time you prescribed the valacyclovir." [In actuality, I had forgotten that I had ordered the PlasMyc six weeks earlier than what I had just told Dr. Brewer.] Dr. Brewer: "Okay. So they were both new." Bob: "Yes."

Dr. Brewer: "So the other question is, is it the combo of those two? See, in other words, that's actually starting to make some sense now. On the PlasMyc, maybe that explains why you got by with a lower dose of the valacyclovir. So the PlasMyc, how many did you take a day?" Bob: "Just one a day." …

The doctor then asked if I'd had any die-off from the valacyclovir and/or the PlasMyc, and I replied that I hadn't had much.

Dr. Brewer next proceeded to talk about an interesting case of his. A female patient — who was around my age, and who Dr. Brewer had been seeing for about 10 years for CFS — was exposed to the mold where she lived when she was 12 years old. However, she was fine until two years later when she fell ill with mono, and she was never well again. That was 41 years ago. She recently tested positive for EBV, and she was now on the valacyclovir.

"One interesting thing about her case, and I've heard several after this, ostensibly she wasn't sick from the mold exposure. But it was pulling down her immune system. See where I'm going with this?" Bob: "Yes." Dr. Brewer: "In other words, the mold didn't seem to be making her sick … and then she's just devastated after this mono. So I think you can get sick from mold; but its predominate factor could be, in many of these cases, it's screwing up the immune system.

"Now we would still like to try and get rid of [your mold], which could be difficult for you, because you seem to react [badly] to everything we try nasally. But we would like to get your immune system back to normal, if we could get rid of the mold. … I mean, we're still dealing with the mold; not very many of my cases respond as adversely as you do to the nasal stuff; it doesn't agree with you very well. But the other thing we're doing is saying, 'Okay, what's active? And let's treat it.' And that's what we've been working on a lot since September.

"Now in your situation, we have pretty definite evidence that EBV is active [and the] HHV-6 is probably active. So in you, it's probably both of them. And then something that we did together on our decision making tree that led into November 5 worked for you.   But it's interesting with you, you did both the transfer factor PlasMyc and the valacyclovir. You did both, so I'm going to want you back on both."

When I asked about dose amounts, the doctor told me I could take as many as two capsules of the PlasMyc daily, and as many as three tablets of the valacyclovir daily. But for now, he wanted me to just go back to the doses I was on leading up to last November 5.

Dr. Brewer: "One of the things that I want you to take home from this … Let's assume that you still have mold toxins inside you, which is a pretty good assumption. And let's assume your immune system is going to be suppressed as long as they are there, and we don't know where the end of that tunnel is. …

Then what in the world will keep EBV and HHV-6 from going active again? If your own God-given immune system is being suppressed by the mold toxins, then when you stop things like PlasMyc and valacyclovir that help control the viruses … you're going back to baseline again.

"If again my assumption is correct: that the mycotoxins are what suppresses your immune system, with emphasis on the gliotoxin. And that's not gone from your body. And how could it be? You don't tolerate the nasal spray very well." …

Bob: "But there was a time we thought [the mold] was all gone, with the mold coming out of my nose." Dr. Brewer: "Right. Right. But based on other patients, I think it's really hard to get rid of. I'm not saying we can't, but I think it's hard. The point is, your immune system is not going to go back to normal overnight. And it's probably going to stay abnormal for the foreseeable future, so we have to try to keep the viruses under control. The point is, you're going to have to stay on this stuff, and you may have to stay on it long term. At least maybe one a day.

"So I think maybe we've stumbled on to the way to get you back pretty healthy again, and it may be the combo of the PlasMyc and the valacyclovir. Now there's going to be some issues about the dosing. Like you said, one or two a day, feel free to play with that. And you've got to watch for die-off and that sort of thing. …

"Now I may have, you know, people start coming in here having stories just as good as yours on the valacyclovir alone. But if I don't, I'm going to be adding the PlasMyc. See, the PlasMyc has activity against both HHV-6A and HHV-6B, EBV, and several other things."

Q. How do some of your other CFS patients get well so quickly, in just three or four months, on the nasal antifungals? Don't they have to detox the mycotoxins out of their system for several months after treatment? **A.** "I don't know. My guess is, it has to do with the genetics of their detoxing. My guess is that you're genetically a slow detox-er and they are not."

Q. Does the transfer factor for Lyme (L-Plus) also work on that same part of the compromised immune system as the PlasMyc? **A.** "I've just reviewed this. The PlasMyc is the most broad spectrum of the ones Researched Nutritionals makes. The one for Lyme, I think it might miss HHV-6A; it might get EBV and [HHV-6] B. But the PlasMyc gets mycoplasma, HHV-6A, HHV-6B, Lyme. It's by far the most broad spectrum one."

Bob: "So if somebody has Lyme, they would probably use the Lyme transfer factor?" Dr. Brewer: "Yes. But if they have the viruses, they might want the PlasMyc. If it's like you're not sure all you have, the PlasMyc would be the most broad spectrum one."

Q. If a person has Lyme, after they start to kill off the mold colonization and detox the mold out of their tissues, when should the Lyme transfer factor come into play? **A:** "It would depend on their die-off reaction. So if they're not having die-off, yes, it would be fine to add that. As you know, both of them can cause die-off. The mold treatment can cause die-off, but also the transfer factor can too. The way I gauge it is, their die-off. If they're *not* having die-off, they can add stuff in pretty quickly. If they are having die-off, they've got to take it pretty slow."

Q. If I could get back to feeling like I did last November 5, that would be helpful for my heart, wouldn't it? **A.** "Yes."

Q. I know the glutathione and methyl Bs can help with detox, but can they cause extra detox? **A.** "Yes. If you take too much, you're going to detox too fast. And that's what happened to you, I think, December 5."

Q. What is the difference between using a nebulizer and the atomizer? (I have a friend whose doctor put her on a nebulizer.) **A.** "The original pharmacy [that we used was the] ASL pharmacy, which is now this Imprimis. ASL told me, [that over] the number of years they had been in business, they had looked at virtually every atomizer/nebulizer on earth. I mean, they looked at everything, and the one that ... had the best patient satisfaction, and seemed to deliver the meds best, according to the ENT doctors, was the NasaTouch [atomizer].

"Now I will say — I'm not sure I want to do anything with you right now on this — but I will say, they've recently come out with a pump spray. … It's just a squirt bottle." Bob: "With the nystatin in it?" Dr. Brewer: "No. That's the problem. But it has amphotericin or itraconazole. Since you had such a nasty time with itraconazole, I would say, 'No, we would not do that.'" The doctor said the reason you can't do the nystatin in a pump spray is because, with the nystatin, you have to start with the powdered drug. It can't be in solution … "but the other two can be in solution.

"So it's called BEG+, then either amphotericin or itraconazole. So they make BEG by itself; BEG with amphotericin, and BEG with itraconazole. They can't do the nystatin because you can't mix it up in solution for a month; they send you the bottle to last you for a month. So BEG is like Bactroban, which is an antibiotic that kills staph, but it doesn't get in your body; it all works topically. The G is gentamicin, which is an antibiotic that kills some other kinds of bacteria that could be in the sinuses. And the E is actually the EDTA; it's the cheating agent that we've had all along, that we used back in the beginning.

"I think the BEG was probably designed by an ENT doc, along the way, that said, 'With my sinus patients, I want to deliver some kind of a biofilm mucus buster along with a couple of antibiotics into the nose,' and they came up with the BEG. ...

"Now they've made the BEG with amphotericin and the BEG with itraconazole. [And] people jump on this like crazy. Why? It takes about 30 seconds a day. Squirt, squirt, and you're done. Now will it work as well as the atomizer? I have no idea. But I have people right now who are doing nothing; they aren't doing anything. And these are people that tolerate it okay. So even if it doesn't work as well as the other one, it's got to be better than nothing, right? We would think. Unless it has zero effect, it's going to work better than nothing. Because with some people, it's just too much of a hassle to mix the nystatin and all that.

"So if we wanted to try to treat your mold in the sinuses again, our options would be ... I don't think we should do itraconazole, because you just got too sick with it. I think our options would be, number one, you could go back to the nystatin, or you could go to the BEG+amphotericin. And there's probably less amphotericin in there than what we had in the atomizer, so I don't think it will burn the nose as much.

"I've started about 20 people on the BEGs, and I've been doing this for about six to eight weeks now, and I haven't had virtually any call-backs complaining. That's so far good news. The reason I don't want to do it right now is, let's do one thing at a time. Let's do everything in our power between the two of us to try and recapture November 5 to December 5. I think you'd agree with me. Whatever you were doing that got you to that spot, we want to get you back there. Hopefully quickly. And it sounds like the big key is the PlasMyc and the valacyclovir."

Q. Has Dr. Brewer ever heard of the NO/ONOO Cycle? If so, what does he think of it? Could mold trigger it? Will treating the mold do away with the NO/ONOO cycle just like the HHV-6? (I ask this because I've read this could be, or is, a big player in fibromyalgia and possibly CFS.)

A. The doctor had heard of the NO/OONO cycle, or "Marty Pall's work" as he called it. And he did think it played a role in fibromyalgia.

Dr. Brewer: "It's kind of involved with inflammation and your antioxidant system. It's a very complex chemical pathway that we all have in us. But what Pall's kind of idea was, that something will trigger … It's a little bit of a horse out of the barn thing. So it's something like emotional stress, or a surgery, or a pregnancy, or something, will trigger the NO/OONO cycle to get out of whack. And then it won't rebalance itself. I don't buy it. I buy that it gets out of whack; I get that, okay?

"My point is, in my opinion, the trigger is an infection. … And probably, when you get EBV, it triggers that cycle to go haywire. … [And] we have evidence now, in almost a 100 patients, of active EBV.

"Now we've had a few people who have never had EBV, so EBV is not the only answer to all of you. There are other issues. There could be Lyme in patients; HHV-6 alone; maybe mycoplasma. ... So there could be a variety of different infections. So I think he's right; the NO/OONO cycle gets out of whack. But I think something set it off. And I think what set it off was an infection.

"But now I think we can take it back a step further. What I think the sequence is: the patient's living or working in a moldy environment; they get a suppressed immune system; they get an active infection, which could be several different things: Lyme, EBV, HHV-6, others. And then their immune system can't get that back under control, and they become chronically ill after that."

Bob: "So basically what you do is, you would go back to the initial mold, infections, and so forth?"

Dr. Brewer: "Yes. The story you laid out before me today I could have almost predicted. The only thing I had forgotten about was, did you start on the PlasMyc? But I mean, if we can get those viruses under control, you should feel better. Well, that's what happened. You get the viruses under control and you feel better.

"The point I'm trying to make over and over and over again to you is, you can't stop this stuff. Now I'm not talking three years from now. I'm talking now. You can't just take this for a month and stop it. It isn't going to work because your immune system is just as bad as it was; well, the PlasMyc probably helped boost it back up. Maybe down the line — but I'll have to give you guidance on this — maybe down the line, you could stop the valacyclovir and maybe the PlasMyc will take care of it. Or vice-versa. We don't know. But like I'm saying, I want to recreate where you were on November 5."

Bob: "That makes a lot of sense." Dr. Brewer: "I'd think you'd like that too. This is the best stretch you've had in years."

On Dr. Lerner, EBV, and the Heart:

Dr. Brewer: "Have you ever seen Dr. Martin Lerner's stuff on EBV and all that?" Bob: "I think I have seen some." Dr. Brewer: "Okay. You might — because I know you spend a lot of time on the Internet — so you might look up … Lerner passed away about a year or so ago [in October 2015], but he was in his 90s. He was this infectious disease doctor in Michigan who did a lot of work on CFS." Bob: "He mentioned the valacyclovir." Dr. Brewer: "Yes, he did. He used a lot of it.

"The interesting thing is, if you look his stuff up, he talks about EBV involving the heart. And he talks about these people — and he's published numerous papers on cardiac involvement with EBV — and they actually have people like you, who had a biopsy of their heart, and they found EBV in their cardiac tissue." Bob: "Wow." Dr. Brewer: "Isn't that cool? Not cool for you. …

"And they found — on their EKGs and ECHOs and so forth — they found, as they had them on the valacyclovir and so forth, their heart improved and went back to normal. So your heart thing even fits.

"And Lerner thinks some of the exercise intolerance and so forth is [that] their heart can't tolerate it. So what Lerner would tell people, when he put them on valacyclovir, is that they should not exercise until they're feeling better. And once they're feeling better, then they're not putting any strain on their heart, and they can start exercising. So this stuff really fits together."

Email to Dr. Brewer on March 14, 2017:
I asked Dr. Brewer about the human anatomy involved with the mold infection. I said that it looked like, from the Internet, that there was a nasal cavity; and also there were three sinus cavities: frontal, ethmoid, and maxillary. And it also looked like the nasal cavity had openings into all three sinus areas.

Q. Is the mold colonization in all three sinus cavities and the nasal cavity? **A.** "Yes, any and all are possible. The ENT literature shows infection can only be in one area or involve them all –- probably kind of random."

Office Visit #25 on August 1, 2017:
Note: Since my last visit, I had continued taking the ImmunoPro and the methyl B vitamins. ~~

In my notes for the doctor:
Starting the 1st of February, I tried to recreate what I'd been taking that led to me to feeling so much better for 30 days beginning last November 5. This meant taking the valacyclovir

and PlasMyc transfer factor again to fight off my reactivated herpes virus infections. My experience was as follows:

a. January 1, 2017: I had already started back on the PlasMyc at one capsule daily.

b. February 1: I started taking one gram of the valacyclovir daily, but I also stopped taking the PlasMyc.

c. March 2: I started back on the PlasMyc transfer factor.

d. March 17: I stopped taking the PlasMyc.

e. March 20: I stopped taking the valacyclovir. I'd been on the PlasMyc and the valacyclovir for 46 days each — and this was the same period as the 46 days I had been on the valacyclovir (and the PlasMyc longer) in the fall of 2016, and which had made me feel so much better. But this time around, instead of feeling better, I became much more ill. [I think at the time I was heavily detoxing — or experiencing *die-off* — from the actions of the PlasMyc and the valacyclovir.]

f. March 26: I went back on the PlasMyc.

g. April 20: I felt that my CFS was fully back for the first time since Thanksgiving 2014, and I felt that my EBV was surging again. So I went back on the valacyclovir for a week, to give a boost to the effect of the PlasMyc.

h. May 1: I started taking probiotics, one 200 billion and one 95 billion daily.

i. May 14: I stopped taking the PlasMyc. That meant I was only on the methylation, glutathione, and (the recently started) probiotic supplements.

j. June 6: I felt good and healthy again, and even better than I had during the previous November (2016) where I'd had 30 good continuous days. I cut my ubiquinol for my heart from 1500 mg daily to 500 mg daily with no ensuing pain. Other than that, I continued to take supplements occasionally for my liver and kidney function, and drugs for sleep.

k. June 11: I sprained my low back and went on pain killers and muscle relaxers. This new development left it hard for me to know where my health was at for sure, as the pain drained my energy and caused me some confusion. Yet, other than my back issue and pain, I continued to feel pretty good.

First the doctor reviewed with me the valacyclovir and PlasMyc I'd been on, as well as my current regimen of supplements.

Dr. Brewer: "So, other than spraining your back, you've done pretty well?" Bob: "Yes. I felt so good on June 9 and 10, maybe I did too much and threw my back out. When I woke up on the 11th, it was really painful. But it was amazing. I mean, I felt healthy again, until I threw my back out. I even felt better than I did last November."

Dr. Brewer: "One concern, somewhat like last November, is what made you better? Obviously, we're glad you're better, except for your back. But we don't know what made you better, and will it hold? Or is this going to be another temporary good stretch? And then the question is, why did you enter the good stretch? There's a couple of factors in there; the valacyclovir and the transfer factor led into this, sort of like they did last fall. But then, of course, last fall you eventually crashed. But was that after you'd stopped them?" Bob: "Yes. After I felt better. And for 30 days, I did pretty well." Dr. Brewer: "And now it's been longer than 30 days?" Bob: "Yes. About seven weeks."

Q: Can a person with Multiple Chemical Sensitivity (MCS) recover if they have the internal live mold and are treated successfully for the mold? **A:** "I think they can. I've heard of cases, and I think I've had some cases, where the symptoms got a lot better. … I look at MCS as a symptom, just like fatigue, or headache, or muscle pain, or joint pain." …

I asked the doctor how he was going to get this mold information out there nationally. He said he and his associates had done that through the four mold papers they had published for free on the Internet. Then he gave a brief description of those papers: "The original, linking CFS to mold; then there's the one about the sinuses, we think mold gets in the sinuses; then there's two on treatment. The first one was on the amphotericin, and the second was on the nystatin."

Q. Have you seen much better results with your patients since you added-in your methyl B vitamins (fall of 2015) and glutathione (mid-2016) protocols along with the antifungal for the mold treatment? Especially with new patients?

A. "Not really. The methyl B-12, if anything, we have seen people feel worse rather than better. Now that's not everybody. So with the methyl B-12, it's like so many things we try, you see three different results. Some people feel worse; some people feel the same, and some people feel better. ...

"The glutathione, I think, is probably tolerated quite a bit better than the methyl B-12. We have seen some people who have seen some improvement on the glutathione, whether it be the NAC form of it or some type of glutathione."

Dr. Brewer said he had even seen patients do better with the IV glutathione. However, he said he'd occasionally seen people have negative reactions to the glutathione, but those negative reactions were a lot less than those seen with the methyl B-12.

Q: How many patients have recovered, significantly or completely, by number or percent, since you began this mold therapy with them back in 2013?

A: "The number that's improved is about the same. One of the issues is, and this is kind of an issue with you. So ... let me give you an example. I just saw one of the two girls this morning, in follow-up. There are these two sisters, so the story is, growing up, and I just reconfirmed this again with one of the girls this morning. These are two sisters that are about a year and a half apart in age.   They're now both in their mid-to-late twenties.

"So, growing up they had bedrooms in their parent's basement. That's where their bedrooms were. That's where they spent most of their time. And this was a wet, damp basement, particularly when it rained, and it had mold down there. So I reconfirmed this morning that, at least the one I saw this morning, she probably started staying in that bedroom in about fifth grade.

"So both of the girls are fine; they have no health problems whatsoever until about 2005 or so. At that point in time, the younger sister was a sophomore in high school. That's basically tenth grade. So she went from fifth grade to tenth grade, living in that basement, sleeping there every night, and felt fine. So in 2005, she comes down with mono. She catches it from another girl at school. And then, within a week later, her sister gets mono.

"So then I see them about 10 years later. I see them in around 2015. Both of them have the same story. They both have a plethora of symptoms: fatigue, headaches, anxiety, brain fog, etc. And they both have the same story: 'We never got over the mono.' They both went to the doctor; they both had a blood test done; they were positive for mono, acute mono on their blood test, and they never recovered.

"[So over the] number of years they lived in that moldy basement, slept and so forth, could [the mold] have interacted with [their immune system] and made it harder to get [the mono] under control?

"So I did the urine test [for toxic mold] on both of them in about 2015, and they were both positive. And they've both done the nasal spray. A little erratically, but they've both done nystatin. And like the one this morning is on it two or three days a week. And it has helped both of them.

"Now the older one was in about six months ago, and I checked her EBV stuff, and it was still pretty high titers on the antibodies. So I went ahead and put her on valacyclovir. Now I have not seen her back in follow-up yet, but she's due in [sometime] in the next couple of months. But her sister told me this morning she's doing pretty well, the older one.

"The younger one we have not done anything with antivirals, and I just checked her EBV stuff this morning. But both of them did pretty well on the nasal alone. They're better than what they were when I first met them. But they're not back to normal. They still have residual symptoms.

"The question I have for myself on those cases, and I don't have the answer, is how much of their symptoms are due to mold alone? How much of their symptoms are due to either EBV, or something like EBV? In other words, some sort of infection that reactivated inside of their system because of the weakened immune system. Or is it a combination of both? Now I have assumed, with many of these cases, like with yours, it may be a combination of both.

"The problem with at least those two, blaming it on the mold alone, why were they okay for at least five years before? ... See, there was a five year period where they slept in that basement every night. We know that the house had mold in it. ... In fact, she told me this morning, mom and dad just sold the house. Before they sold the house, they had to get the entire basement gutted, and remodel the whole thing, because of the water leaks and the mold. And they found black mold everywhere down there. So we know that they had mold in the basement.

"But from fifth grade to tenth grade, she's fine. Until she gets mono. But my initial treatment from 2015 going forward was only nasal spray, and it worked pretty well. Now it didn't make her completely 100% well, but she probably has about a 50% to 60% reduction in her symptoms. But she had not had any reduction in her symptoms, with anything else, over a period of 10 years.

"So they're a classic example of, how much of this is due to mold? How much of it's due to, in their case, EBV? Or is it both?

"Now obviously the approach I've taken with the older girl that I saw back a few months ago is, we're going to try and treat for both. We've got her on the valacyclovir and the nasal stuff. So we'll see how things go with her. Again, the sister told me she's doing pretty well.

"So when you talk about mold people getting better, it's more complicated in cases than just mold.

"It's the same thing with Lyme disease. Somebody had been exposed to mold, and then they got a tick bite, and they got Lyme disease; then we treat the Lyme with antibiotics. Then how much of the symptoms are due to Lyme, and how much of it's due to the mold?

"That's kind of a long-winded answer to that, but it kind of applies to you. How much of it is due, in your case, maybe to the EBV and the weakened immune system, versus how much of that's due to the mold. In other words, we have direct symptoms due to mold, where somebody's living in a moldy place and gets sick immediately. And then we have indirect symptoms, of which I think one of the biggest indirect things is the immune system suppression. Which would not surprise you."

Note: Dr. Nathan says that Dr. Shoemaker's work has shown that not everybody who is exposed to the same toxic mold environment will get sick. Dr. Nathan believes this is because everyone has their own individual biochemical component that decides their reaction to any toxic mold exposure. This means that if two people get exposed to the same toxic mold environment and only one gets sick, you can't use the one who didn't fall ill to discredit the validity of the illness of the one who did get sick. ~~

Q. I have a friend in California [Steve] who is following the doctor's mold protocol, and he has also been using supplements like glutathione, on his own, in what he calls a *liposomal delivery system*. After three and a half months, he says he's about 70% well again. What does Dr. Brewer think about using the liposomal supplements?

A. "The liposomal delivery system is very interesting." The doctor said you can get about everything in a liposomal supplement. It was particularly good with vitamin C, as vitamin C was not easily absorbed. "It is an exciting new area of drug delivery and supplement delivery." He said the glutathione, by the way, was poorly absorbed. The NAC was absorbed pretty well with the acetal group; and the ImmunoPro, as whey protein, was also well absorbed. And the liposomal glutathione was markedly superior to regular glutathione.

Q. If you cure the mold, do the stiff red blood cells seen in CFS go back to normal? **A.** "Yes, it's possible."

Q: Should we do another mold test? Or maybe we should just wait and see if I relapse again?

A. The doctor said waiting for a relapse in my health would probably be best before doing another mold test. If I relapse and the EBV comes back, then the mold is probably still a problem. If I reach that point, I should start back on the valacyclovir and the transfer factor PlasMyc; do a mold test and send it in; and if the mold isn't gone, he'll put me back on an intranasal antifungal. He also told me (as he did last visit) they were now using a nasal spray for the BEG+amphotericin and the BEG+itraconazole, but it was not available with the nystatin.

Bob: "Can it be possible that the mold is gone, but I still have a problem with the recurring EBV?" Dr. Brewer: "Yes. But it's unlikely the mold is gone. … I think it's very difficult, possibly impossible, although I'm not quite there yet, to get rid of the mold out of the sinuses. So what I tell people with the nasal spray, we're trying to either reduce the amount or eradicate it. Now eradicate it means we get rid of every last stitch of it. I'm not sure we can eradicate it, but I do think we can reduce the amount that's in the sinuses. Which means that people will probably need to stay on maintenance nasal spray, but that could be something like once a week or twice a week." …

Bob: "Have you ever seen people that were cured, and then they came back later and had had a relapse?" Dr. Brewer: "Yes. With an elevated urine test." Bob: "Is that common?" Dr. Brewer: "Yes, it is. Most of my people have had to go back on the nasal spray." The doctor then gave me a good example of this with one of his patients.

Bob: "This is not encouraging, really." Dr. Brewer: "I understand that."

Bob: "So, when somebody does relapse, do they go back on a full dose until they feel better?" Dr. Brewer: "Yes." This was in cases where the patient hadn't ever experienced any die-off in their earlier nasal therapy. In such cases, the doctor put them back on a full dose of the nasal antifungals to begin with; and then, maybe in two or three months, they could start cutting that full dose down to a maintenance dose. He added that the maintenance doses seemed to work.

Bob: "What about the others?" Dr. Brewer: "Sometimes they go back on a smaller dose. It kind of varies."

Bob: "What do you mean when you say die-off?" Dr. Brewer: "When they do the spray, they feel worse. Like if they do it too many days in a row. It's like when you felt worse doing it. That's what we're calling die-off." Bob: "Is that mold die-off?" Dr. Brewer: "Yes. That's what we think." …

Bob: "So when I was on the nystatin, and had the dead mold come out of my nostrils, that was die-off?" Dr. Brewer: "Part of it, yes."

Dr. Brewer then summarized what we'd just discussed for me to do should I relapse again. He specifically added that, if I did go back on an antifungal, not to begin it too close to when I started back on the antivirals. I assumed this was to keep me from having mold die-off on top of viral die-off.

Dr. Brewer: "Anyway, for the moment, I think we got a pretty reasonable plan. You're doing okay, except you sprained your back. But for the moment, you're doing okay. And let's hope it continues. If it doesn't, I think we need to have a strategic plan of what to do." Bob: "Okay. It sounds like we got it." …

While Dr. Brewer was ordering a mold testing kit for me to take with me when I left, I said: "I've sent some of this [mold] information off to Florida. No response. I sent some of this information out to California. I got two people interested. One of those guys is almost completely healed; the other one's still struggling. But I was trying to figure out, how come nobody's interested in this?" Dr. Brewer: "If you find out, will you tell me?"

Bob: "The guy from California told me, he said it was presented to the support group out there, and he said none of the people are interested because they don't believe they've been exposed to mold." Dr. Brewer: "But it could go back to their parent's house; it could've been in their dorm room in college. I've got over five cases right now that were exposed in their dorm room in college."

Bob: "So the exposure doesn't have to be right before you get sick?" Dr. Brewer: "No. It could have been 30 years ago. Because it gets in the sinuses and makes a home in the sinuses." Bob: "So symptoms may appear years later?" Dr. Brewer: "Years later. So that's the key. That's what most people don't understand. It could be an old exposure. ... I have people that were probably exposed when they were a kid."

<u>Chapter Five: Treatment Protocols?</u>

My California friend, Steve, has also been on this journey of healing from mold exposure. His medical diagnosis was for ME (Myalgic Encephalomyelitis), not CFS.

Steve began his journey by taking liposomal glutathione twice a day for two weeks before he had his *Mycotoxin Panel* done with RealTime Labs back in October 2016. His test results showed that he was positive for infection in all four mycotoxin categories. Then, in the first four months of his antifungal mold treatment on the amphotericin B, he reported his functionality had gone from 25% to 70%. The treatment also allowed him to get out of assisted living and into his own apartment.

In an update in June 2020, I got a call from Steve. Since October 2016, Steve had continued on the nasal antifungal amphotericin. He also continued to be tested for mold toxins in his urine, having tests done again in 2017, 2018, and 2019. Steve reported that he got completely well in June 2019, so he had been healthy again for a year by the time of this particular call. As such, he'd been going to the gym; going hiking in the mountains; etc. But while his mold toxin levels had mostly come down by mid-2019, his test numbers had remained elevated enough to where they still showed him as being positive for mold infection.

However, on this June 2020 date — which was a year following his mid-2019 mold toxin test — Steve told me that three of his four mold toxins, in a new mycotoxin test, had finally come down to zero. This meant he was finally getting the mold toxins completely flushed out of his tissues. As for the fourth mold toxin, Steve didn't seem to think its toxin level was all that high. So for Steve, it took him about a year after he felt much better before his output of mold toxins substantially dropped.

In what follows, I've shown my friend Steve's mold treatment protocol first, as he told it to me, and which was patterned after Dr. Brewer's treatment protocol. And then, after that, I've shown what I personally used.

<u>Warning</u>: Please note that I didn't take everything mentioned below all of the time. Also, patients should *only* take these drugs and supplements, in either individual doses or in combinations, while under the supervision and care of a knowledgeable medical doctor. That's what Steve and I did. ~~

For mold treatment, Steve took what he called his "Triple Play," while I took these things individually:

a. One spoonful (500 mg) of physician formulated Core Med Science liposomal glutathione (made of the Japanese Setria brand, which is "China-Free"); and which also contains 500 mg of a phosphatidylcholine complex. This is available from: https://www.amazon.com.

- I used one scoop of the ImmunoPro powder every other day.

b. Amphotericin, 5 mg capsules, from Cascade Specialty Pharmacy (800-822-2029). Steve emptied one capsule, mixed with [the EDTA dissolved in a] saline solution, into a NeilMed Sinus Rinse bottle; then he squirted one half of the bottle contents into each nostril twice a day.

  - I don't recall exactly what I took, but according to my notes and Dr. Brewer's third paper on the antifungal intranasal therapy, in the end it *appears* that I took: the EDTA in the morning; and one capsule containing 50,000 units [5 mg] of the nystatin mixed with 5 ml [0.17 oz] of distilled water later in the day; and I used the NasaTouch atomizer to deliver both of these agents into my nasal passages. I started out doing one dose every two days, and I ended-up doing one dose every three days due to the die-off reaction I had in-between doses.

c. Methyl B vitamins: One spoonful (1/2 teaspoon / 2.5 ml dose) of Quantum Nutrition Labs brand "Max Stress B" supplement, which contains methylated B vitamins in a liquid extract. See: http://qnlabs.com/max-stress-b.html.

  - I eventually settled on taking 250 micrograms of methyl B-12 and 200 micrograms of methyl folate once every three days.

Because the mold therapy and its detox can apparently cause constipation, my California friend took four things every day that helped him with elimination:

a. Lactulose prescription medication in the morning, with lactulose being a non-absorbable sugar used in the treatment of constipation.

b. One teaspoon unheated sea salt in the morning.

c. Docusate Sodium (stool softener), 250 milligram capsule at bedtime; and OJC Organic Juice Cleanse Plus [a super food] at one teaspoon every morning.

- I varied what I took for constipation, using: Naturade Stool Softener Laxative, Nature's Life Herbs and Prunes, MiraLAX, and organic prune juice.

Because the mold detox process can make the bodily systems too acidic, my California friend took (a) mineral supplementation, and (b) half a teaspoon of baking soda per day. This combination put his pH back in its normal range.

- I took nothing for my body pH.

Finally, my California friend said it's practical and helpful to do some of the following in order to make the whole process smoother:

a. Vitamin C (available from https://qnlabs.com).

b. R-Lipoic acid (one capsule twice a day).

- • I took 100 mg of the Doctor's Best R-Lipoic-Acid with the ImmunoPro glutathione supplement.

c. NAC (one capsule twice a day).
- • I (briefly) took 600 mg of Jarrow brand NAC Sustain daily.

d. Probiotic — with as many strains as possible; the more billion CFU (or colony-forming units) the better — to help with gut issues (https://qnlabs.com has a good probiotic).
- • I took high-CFU, refrigerated probiotics bought from my local health food store.

e. Pectin: one or two capsules, with meals, twice a day.

f. Bentonite clay (which is used to help eliminate mycotoxins from the intestinal tract): you open the capsule into a drink; and it's to be taken twice a day, with meals.
- • I took one capsule daily of the Redmond Clay bentonite clay, and I alternated that with periods where I took one charcoal capsule daily.*

g. Evening primrose oil.
- • I took this supplement at times as well.

* Note: Dr. Brewer had given me a handout early on that talked about *mycotoxin binders,* which were substances that bound mycotoxins in the GI tract and prevented their reabsorption back into the blood stream. It said activated charcoal worked on all toxins; Bentonite clay and zeolite clay only bound aflatoxins; and a few other possibilities were Chitosan, Glucomannan, Pectin, Cholestyramine, and probiotics like Align and Culturelle.~~

Robert Roy

Advance Note: In one definition, homeopathic medicines are said to be minuscule amounts of therapeutic substances, such as those taken from plants, that are first highly diluted in grain alcohol; and then again diluted in a mixture of water and alcohol. At each stage of the dilution, the mixture is vigorously shaken to assure the therapeutic effect of the medicine. ~~

<u>Warning</u>:

Before going on to the next section, I would advise upfront that unless you are experienced in their use, I would not use any of the homeopathic medicines listed below (or similar type ones), except under the guidance of an experienced health care practitioner. Otherwise, questions will arise with their use: which homeopathic liquid do I use for which problem; how many drops do I take; etc.? In my experience, just taking a few drops too many of a homeopathic medicine can sometimes cause a severe physical adverse reaction. (I personally never take more than 10 drops of any homeopathic.)

In one of his radio interviews with Dr. Brewer, Dr. Nathan mentioned how he used homeopathic drainage remedies — for the liver, kidneys, and lymphatic system — with his mold patients to help with their bodily detoxification processes. I used similar homeopathic products myself, and these were made by the company Apex Energetics. Some of the ones I have used are:

a. Futureplex Antitox D-3 LVR-DRN (liver drain)
b. Futureplex Antitox A13 DTX-LIVER
c. Futureplex Antitox D-5 KDNY-DRN (kidney drain)
d. Futureplex Antitox A12 DTX-KIDNEY
e. Futureplex Antitox D-8 LNG-DRN (lung drain)
f. Futureplex Antitox D-7 LYMPH-DRN (lymph drain)
g. Futureplex Antitox A-14 DTX-Lymph (detox lymph)
h. Futureplex Antitox A-2 Gentle Drainage
i. Futureplex Antitox N-3 Exchem
j. Futureplex Antitox B1 Acute Rescue

After reading Dr. Nathan's book *Toxic,* I began using two other homeopathic remedies:
a. Deseret Biologicals Systemic Drainage
b. Deseret Biologicals Detox 1

Chapter Six: Colloidal Silver

Office Visit #26 with Dr. Brewer on May 30, 2018:

On this date, it had been about 10 months since my last appointment. I had been scheduled to see Dr. Brewer the previous February, but unforeseen circumstances had caused that appointment to be cancelled.

In my notes for the doctor:
a.   June 8, 2017: As I had reported last visit, on this date I had felt much better, even healthy again.
b.   July 10: after recovering from a back sprain from last June, my sleep meds quit working. I had been on those meds off-and-on for years, and they were 1.0 mg of clonazepam (17 years) and 125 mg of amitriptyline (6 years).
c.   July 10 to October 9: I tapered off my sleep meds for the next three months. [Why I hadn't reported that I had started this tapering off to the doctor on my last visit is beyond me. He might have been able to save me some real miscry if I had.]
d.   October 10: the next day, after stopping all my sleep meds, I started having severe liver pain and severe insomnia. I wondered if I was detoxing my old sleep meds.

e.   November 9: Even with severe liver pain, my liver enzymes tested normal, and an MRI showed no change in my fatty liver and no other liver problems.

f.   Late November: besides the continuing severe liver pain, I developed diarrhea (one watery stool per day), and I had a recurring rash over my liver.

g.   December 1: My primary care doctor told me they had sent a referral to Dr. J., the liver specialist who I'd seen before, but so far I have not heard back from Dr. J.'s office.

h.   December 20: My liver pain had started to ease by this time, and a gastroenterologist in Lawrence that I saw put me back on 50 mg of the amitriptyline that I used to take. With both these events, I started to sleep a little better, but only during the day.

i.   Early April: My mind became clearer.

j.   Early May: my sleep worsened; my diarrhea worsened; the long recurring rash over my liver, when it appeared, stayed around longer, and I started having kidney pain.

k.   Mid-May: I saw an acupuncturist. My sleep improved; my liver pain dropped to mild; I started sleeping during the night, and my watery stools went back to once a day.

Dr. Brewer: "It's possible that going off the two sleeping meds, or the two medications that you were taking at bedtime, it could have been withdrawal. You're calling it detox, but it's kind of the same thing with withdrawal. Benzodiazepines, clonazepam, for

17 years — that's really, really hard to get off of, for anybody. Some people can't do it. They can go down, but they can't get off.

"Since it happened the following day, I'm pretty sure it was a withdrawal thing. But it shouldn't last that long. It might even last a month or two. … I think the next day, and at least a few weeks thereafter, it was withdrawal. Whether that's still going on now, I'm not sure."

Bob: "I just kind of got the feeling that it started some other kind of detox." Dr. Brewer: "It might have. But the fact that it was the next day. I mean, it wasn't like a week later. It's like your body's going, 'Where's my clonazepam?' Even though it was a lower dose, you did it right. I mean, I'm not critical of how you did it. I think you did it right. Your body's going, 'Bob, where's my medicines tonight? I'm going to rebel.'

"Are you still on the small dose [of the amitriptyline that the gastroenterologist] put you on?" Bob: "Yes. But not the clonazepam." Dr. Brewer: "Yes, just the amitriptyline. The amitriptyline's much less habit forming. This could have been all clonazepam. And the one that's really, really hard to get off of, this clonazepam. It's in that benzodiazepine category. So now that you're off of it, see if you can stay off of it. I'm okay with the amitriptyline. And that's a small dose.

Bob: "Have other people tried to get off the clonazepam and had this kind of reaction?" Dr. Brewer: "Several had to go to the emergency room. I had one guy that went off cold turkey and ended up in the emergency room. He had to go back on it. He was hallucinating and everything else. Now he went off from a higher dose. …

"I do think you should see a liver specialist because of your fatty liver. I don't know, all this pain over your liver and so forth, because your liver enzymes are okay; and your MRI showed you [still have] fatty liver. Maybe to get a baseline on your fatty liver, and is there anything else to be done for that."

Then I had some questions about other prominent CFS doctors who were, or might be, working with mold in CFS.

Q. On a website [that is no longer available], it said: "Dr. Paul Cheney, Dr. [Kenny] De Meirleir and Dr. [Daniel] Peterson are now using tests for mycotoxins as part of their diagnostics protocol for ME/CFS." Did Dr. Brewer know if this was true about Dr. Peterson and Dr. De Meirleir? **A.** Dr. Brewer had not heard anything on this. [I was to see later that Dr. Peterson was listed on RealTime Lab's list of health care practitioners who specialize in mold and mycotoxin Treatment.]

Q. I asked the doctor if he had heard the following quote from Dr. Nancy Klimas: "With the help of the expert training of the American Academy of Environmental Medicine, we are now testing and treating people with mycotoxin poisoning. It is wonderful to see people getting better!"

A. Dr. Brewer had not heard of this quote, but he said: "I find it interesting that Klimas is showing some interest, too. And I might mention, I gave a talk at the international Lyme meetings in November. And a lot of the Lyme treating doctors test for mycotoxins. I mean, a lot of them." [These meetings had been put on by the International Lyme and Associated Disease Society.]

Note 1: It is apparent from a radio interview of Dr. Brewer — done on December 15, 2014, and for a time posted on the website https://www.voiceamerica.com — that one of the interviewers, Dr. Jacob Teitelbaum, was also prescribing antifungal treatments for his patients at the time. Dr. Teitelbaum is a well known fibromyalgia doctor and the author of several books on health and medicine, and who once had a medical practice near Baltimore, Maryland. He nows lives in Kailua-Kona, Hawaii. He is also listed on RealTime Lab's list of health care practitioners who specialize in Mold and Mycotoxin Treatment.

Note 2: About two months after this office visit, I had an email exchange with Dr. Sarah Myhill, a CFS specialist who has her medical office in Wales. Dr. Myhill told me that — as with Dr. Brewer — she was looking into treating patients for intranasal mold infections. However, she was using the intranasal Lugol's iodine instead of the intranasal antifungal medicines that Dr.

Brewer had been using. In addition, it was *my impression* that this was not as major a focus for her as it was for Dr. Brewer.

Dr. Myhill would go on to include information about two of Dr. Brewer's published papers on toxic mold on the website at: h t t p s : / / d r m y h i l l . c o . u k / w i k i / Chronic_Fungal_Infection_as_a_cause_of_disease:_the_toxicity _of_mycotoxins. ~~

Note: In an office visit on December 11, 2023, I told Dr. Brewer that Dr. Myhill now had links to his papers on her website.

Dr. Brewer: "So I was supposed to go to England in June of 2020, to give a talk at a CFS conference in London, and I had done everything except arrange for my flight — my wife was going to go with me — and you know what happened in 2020 [Covid]. So I had exchanged a bunch of emails with Dr. Myhill, you know, 'We're so excited you're coming' and so forth. I felt sorry for her. She was optimistic up until the last minute that it was going to occur, but I finally had to, by April or May of 2020, I said, 'I'm not coming.' …

Bob: "You know, I sent her an email a couple of years ago, and I asked her if she was interested in your stuff, and she said to send her some information, so I emailed her …" Dr. Brewer: "She contacted me probably in the fall of 2019 and invited me to be a speaker on mold. Maybe you were the genesis of all that."
~~

Dr. Brewer and I then moved on to discussing the other questions I had for the doctor.

Q. Since I hadn't heard back from the liver specialist about an appointment, would Dr. Brewer go ahead and also give me a recommendation to see Dr. J.? **A.** Yes.

A discussion followed. I said that I read that the RealTime Labs test had increased the various mycotoxins they tested for in their four groups. This led to our talking about the RealTime Labs test and another newer, comparable one from the Great Plains Lab [now Mosaic Diagnostics]. Dr. Brewer said he still likes the RealTime Labs test best. And he said he thought we ought to do another mold test on me as well. I told the doctor that I still had a mold test kit at home that I could use for that.

Q: I corresponded briefly with science writer Julie Rehmeyer, who had written a book about her own experience with CFS and toxic mold called *Through the Shadowlands*. She said Dr. Brewer's work would never be taken seriously because the doctor didn't use a control group, which meant that most academic researchers wouldn't pay much attention to it. Since you used a control group on the mold testing, did she mean you didn't use a control group in giving your patients the nasal antifungals — like in giving some patients a nasal placebo?

A: "There have been two criticisms — they're valid criticisms — in that, in our original paper on CFS and mold, we had a control group, but it was a historical control group. In other words, it wasn't a concomitant match control group. ... So that's a valid criticism. But it's the only control we have. We don't have any others. Nobody's wanted to fund a study like that.

"And then, on the nasal-type fungal therapy, that was all just treating patients. We've told people, on these criticisms, they're valid, but we've never said these were *case-controlled studies*. We've said these were *observational studies*. We wondered if mold could be an issue, and if you treated it, could [patients] improve? And so, this is what we observed. Observation studies are not perfect, but they're better than nothing."

Note: Dr. Brewer said elsewhere that the "historical control group" he used came from a study done about five years before he published his first mold paper. This study had been done by RealTime Labs, and for this control group RealTime Labs hadn't eliminated people who *might* have been exposed to toxic mold.

~~

Dr. Brewer: "There is going to be a treatment symposium for doctors in Dallas, in August of this year, on mold treatment. I'm giving one of those talks. There's like 10 or 12 speakers. Dr. Nathan's going to be there speaking. ... That'll probably be online." Bob: "Is that another RealTime thing?" Dr. Brewer: "Yes. RealTime is sponsoring the meeting." …

I told Dr. Brewer that I still had a mold test kit at home that I had got from him last August. I asked, if I did another mold test, could I use that one without any problem? He said it was still good to use and to send in.

Dr. Brewer: "So let me tell you about an interesting new development with the nasal spray. … So at the meetings I was at, the Lyme meetings last fall, my talk was on mold. And mold in general, and maybe its possible relationship with Lyme, and so forth. And a lot of the talk [and emphasis] was on the [nasal] antifungals, which is what I'm going to emphasize in my talk in Texas, too.

"So I did meet a gentleman afterward, after my talk, who came up to me — he's a microbiologist — and he was telling me about a new nasal spray that they have developed. He did some of the background microbiological work on it, and then he worked with a compounding pharmacy in Massachusetts to make the product. So this is a colloidal silver nasal spray.

"Now the first thing they did were some test tube studies, where they took a bunch of different molds, as well as bacteria. So they took molds like Aspergillus and so forth, a variety of different molds; and they also took bacteria — staph [staphylococcus], strep [Streptococcus], etc. — in the test tube; and they exposed them to increased concentrations of colloidal silver. And then they looked at, where did they get a 100% kill, or would they get a 100% kill? If so, at what concentration? What was the minimal concentration that they got that? So they found the concentration where, at that concentration, or above that concentration, they got a 100% kill on everything. All the bacteria and all the molds.

"So then they went to a compounding pharmacy in Massachusetts and [had this made] into a nasal spray. Now it's a little like — just the functionality in the nasal spray — it's a little like the BEG nasal spray. It's a pump sprayer — instead of the little machine, the NasaTouch [atomizer] — it's a pump sprayer.

"Now they've done two additional things with the nasal spray. They've added two additional things to it, and they're both biofilm busters. One is the original biofilm buster we've all been using, the EDTA. So it's got the EDTA in it, which is the E in the BEG. And it's got another biofilm buster called Mucolox. Mucolox was new to me, and I don't know a lot about it. I've talked to the pharmacist.

"So basically the product is a triple combination. It's got the colloidal silver, which of course is the workhorse. The issue was, they weren't sure if the colloidal silver — colloidal silver's a very small molecule; colloidal just means it's suspended in water — and so they weren't sure if it would penetrate biofilm or not. No one really knows if it will penetrate biofilm. But they decided that, to give it the best chance of working, to go ahead and make it with the biofilm busters. So again, it's got two biofilm busters: the EDTA and the Mucolox. And the colloidal silver.

"Now they didn't come out with this until late summer; I didn't hear about it until late November, and I didn't even talk to the pharmacy until December. So in December, I had a pretty significant discussion with the pharmacy about how much does this stuff cost, and how many times a day do you use it, and how do I order it for my patients, etc.?

"So I've had a few patients that started in late December, and then a lot of patients have started since the first of the year. I probably have between 50 and 75 patients who have been on it. Because I see my patients usually every six months, I have very little face-to-face feedback. One feedback we do have is, we have not had anyone call in with side effects. No one. Not a single person has called back and said, 'Oh gosh, I'm having nose bleeds; it's burning my nose,' or anything like that. We haven't had any of that, which is encouraging.

"Now we've had a couple of people that I've seen where it looks like it's working very well. So I would say we're optimistic that this is going to be a good treatment. It might be better than what we've used before. It might even be better than the amphotericin and so forth. But we just don't know yet.

"The pharmacy, even when I talked to them in December, said that the customers and the doctors were really extremely excited about how well it was working. ... Now here almost any time, I'll be seeing a lot of these people back. Because, if I started people in December and January, I'm going to start seeing my six month appointments this summer.

"Now I've already seen two or three. I've had one lady from Lawrence — this is an interesting story; she lives down south of Lawrence — who got completely well. This is back in about 2015. She got completely well on the amphotericin nasal spray, and then she eventually went off of it.

"She did well for about a year, and then she relapsed. And so I saw her back in December, and all of her symptoms had come back. Now she had been off all nasal spray for about a year or so, probably since sometime in 2016. And so I talked to her about going back on the same old nasal spray she did before, which worked, or trying the new one. And she finally, because the pump spray device is easier, she decided to try the new one.

"So I saw her back about two weeks ago; and it took about two months for it to kind of, quote, 'kick in'; and by the end of March she was about 70% improved. Not a 100%, but a lot, lot better. And then, unfortunately, she had to suddenly go out of town because of family illness. And she was about ready to reorder when she got called out of town, so she didn't get to reorder it. So while she was out of town, she was off of it for three weeks. And she completely crashed in three weeks off of it. And went all the way back down again in three weeks. And then, when I saw her a couple of weeks ago, she'd been back on it for about two weeks and was still feeling crummy. But of course, it had only been two weeks.

"Now we've had a phone call — I haven't seen this lady yet, but she's called in — and it sounds like she had a similar experience, where she took it for two months; crashed [while] off of it, and now she's back on it.

"So I was hopeful, because this had a 100% kill in the test tube, this wouldn't need to be a very long course of therapy. So right now, doctor doesn't know how long the course of therapy is going to have to be on this one. But like I say, the early results look good. Hopefully, I'll have quite a bit more feedback by the time I go to the meeting in Texas. Early on, things look good. No side effects and probably working quite well."

Bob: "So you still have a lot of people relapsing?" Dr. Brewer: "If they go off. Now there's two ways to look at it. The problem with the relapse is, is it due to the mold or not? Now in the case of that lady from Lawrence, it's pretty obvious. ... But other cases, let's say [they've] been off for a year, year and a half, and they relapse again. Was it the mold or is it not the mold? Now the urine test can help in that regard. There's two ways to look at a relapse. A return of symptoms, when they're off of it; and then the urine values go back up.

"So what I suggest with you is, let's get the urine test, which you've already got the kit at home. Let's get the urine test and see if you still have elevated values. And if you do, my suggestion would be to take the colloidal silver nasal spray.

"So the name of the pharmacy we've been using that has it is called Hopkinton, and they're in Massachusetts. So that's who makes it. So what we do, we just fax them an order and they'll contact you directly. So if your levels come back elevated, we'll fax you in an order to Hopkinton. [As mentioned earlier, Hopkinton was bought out by PD Labs in Cedar Park, TX, and can be found at: https://pdlabsrx.com.]

"Now the colloidal silver is two squirts. Again, it's a pump sprayer, like the BEG, so it's two squirts in each nostril three times a day. If you forget the middle one, don't worry about it. At least get it in twice a day. A bottle of it costs about $120, but the bottle will last about two months. So it's about $60 a month. And we don't know how many months you have to be on it. … I was hoping to be able to take people off after a month or two, but now I'm a little gun-shy after hearing a couple of these stories."

Bob: "Before you said you had a lot of patients that relapsed and had gone back on a maintenance dose." Dr. Brewer: "Yes. And those people are still doing well. My people that did really well, even on the amphotericin, and they're still on maintenance, are doing well. I have a young woman who lives south of Wichita. She does maintenance about one or two days a week, and she's on amphotericin. I told her about the colloidal silver, but we both decided that — unless it's a permanent fix, to get rid of the mold permanently, and it might be, we just don't know how long you'll have to use it — she might as well just stay on what she's on because it works great. And it's not that big a hassle to do it one day a week. So I still have people on maintenance who are still doing fine.

"And so the colloidal silver may end up to be like that; it [may end up being] maintenance as well. But we don't know. It may take a year or two to figure that out.

"So the question is, is it going to be not as good as an antifungal like the amphotericin; the same, or better? Time will tell. If you base it on the test tube studies, it ought to be better, based on how dramatic the kill effect was in the test tube.

"The other thing is, mold makes spores; and there's probably spores up in the sinuses, and there is some suggestion the colloidal silver may be able to kill the spores."

Bob: "I'm still doing somewhat better." Dr. Brewer: "Yes. You were doing pretty well until you went off the sleeping meds. And again, I'm not critiquing you. I think it was a valiant thing to try." Bob: "The meds weren't working. So, I don't have the virus effects; I have about half my energy back; about half my strength; about half my mind. So it's hard for me to tell, though, with all this other stuff, along with my liver, just ..." Dr. Brewer: "Right. Maybe your liver will check out great. I'm pretty encouraged, because the blood test and the MRI looked okay. ...

Then the doctor changed subjects: "So let me tell you about this supplement." He said he would email me the address on where to get it.

"It's called PEA. So this is a molecule that is inside of us normally; it's a normal molecule inside the body. We all have it inside of us. It appears that its role, inside the body, is to counter-balance and diminish inflammation. Which would be a very good thing for somebody like you. Now the inflammation could be anywhere. It could be in your brain; it could be in your liver, your muscles, your joints, arthritis. It could be anywhere. … But it could counter some of the bad effects of the mold. I'm mainly telling you this because of your liver, but I'm just telling you the brand story first.

"The lady who discovered it is a biochemist in Italy. She had already won the Nobel prize for discovering a different molecule, and then she discovered PEA and how it works. And that it's an anti-inflammatory. Again, it's a natural substance we all have in our body.

"It's been shown to help with fibromyalgia, migraines, chronic joint pain, chronic muscle pain, chronic nerve pain, etc. I'm taking it, and I'm healthy. Why am I taking it? Because in a mouse model it prevents Alzheimers. And it's dramatic. I don't want to wait until I'm 80 and figure out I should have started [on it] back when I was in my 60s. I have my wife on it. It has no side effects. …

"Now I found one paper, I believe this was in an animal model, where it reversed the inflammation in fatty liver. So that's the reason I'm telling you about it. Now it might be good for your brain, and your achiness, and other parts of you too. It's suggested that it would help fatty liver, because what happens with fatty liver is, the fat accumulation is fine; it's not the end of the world. Unless it starts causing inflammation. And it can lead to cirrhosis.   So if you can quell and calm down that inflammation, that might be a good thing. And in this one animal thing, that was pretty dramatic. …

"It's not been real popular in the United States, and I don't know why. The research on it is fairly new, and it's been mainly out of Europe, so that may be the key to it. But it's really a neat product, and there's some fantastic research out of Europe on it."
…

Bob: "Have you ever heard of this thing CIRS?" Dr. Brewer: "Chronic Inflammatory Response Syndrome." Bob: "Is that part of something that Shoemaker …" Dr. Brewer: "Shoemaker created the term. He talks about inflammation due to the mold. So that's why I'm saying, indirectly it could help with mold. It doesn't have anything to do with mold directly; it's just that this is a natural anti-inflammatory. But if mold is creating inflammation, obviously the best thing would be to get rid of the mold. But if mold is creating inflammation — or if other things, like in your liver, fat could be creating inflammation — this doesn't care where the inflammation is, it quells the inflammation. …

"You're a lot better than you were two or three years ago." Bob: "I know. And I'm very thankful for that."

We summarized the visit: take the RealTime Labs test again; and if my mycotoxin numbers are still high, consider taking the intranasal colloidal silver.

Bob: "So I remember in maybe 2015 and when I was retested, all my numbers for the mold had gone up three times higher, and you said you thought that it was detox." Dr. Brewer: "Right. But see, this time it wouldn't be, because you're not on any specific therapy. Back then, I believe you were on something for the mold. This time you're not. So it'll be a true reading of what you're like today, because you're not doing any specific treatment. When you're doing treatment, then the question is, are you flushing more toxins out because you're treating it? But that wouldn't be the case this time."

Here is the link that Dr. Brewer later emailed me as to where I could order the PEA (or Palmitoylethanolamide): https://vitalitus.com/product/pea/?ref=3.

As to dosage, the website says "the recommended dosage [is] two capsules per day … [but if recommended by a physician,] in some cases our customers see a benefit from consuming 4 capsules a day for two to three weeks when starting a PEA regimen."

And from my notes: For best results in taking the PEA, it is recommended you take it with foods containing a small amount of oils or healthy fats (e.g. dairy, eggs, bacon, butter, steak, Italian salad dressing, coconut oil, fish oil capsules, etc.).

<u>Letter from Dr. Brewer dated June 12, 2018:</u>
Dr. Brewer wrote: "I have received your most recent urine mycotoxin results (copy enclosed). As you can see, you were

positive for all four mycotoxins. The ochratoxin was quite high, and the gliotoxin was moderately high.

"I think we should go ahead and proceed with the colloidal silver nasal spray as we had discussed. If you would like us to send in a prescription, just let us know and we will send that in to Hopkinton Drug in Massachusetts."

However, I was struggling to understand these mycotoxin numbers. My ochratoxin ppb had soared from 2.8 in 2013 to 9.508 in 2018; my aflatoxin had gone from zero in 2013 to 1.512 in 2018; my trichothecene had actually dropped slightly, from 0.38 in 2013 to .037 in 2018; and my gliotoxin levels rose somewhat, from 2.76 ppb when they were first tested in 2016 to 3.36 ppb now in 2018.

I continued to believe (falsely, as it would later turn out) that since Thanksgiving 2014 the mold in my nasal passages was dead and gone, and that now I was simply continuing to detox mold toxins out of my tissues.

Still, the aflatoxin numbers were puzzling. I mean, how could my aflatoxin numbers have gone from zero to 1.512 over the last five years when I had not been living in a toxic mold environment? The only answer I could come up with was, in 2013 with my first mycotoxin test, for whatever reason the aflatoxin toxins weren't showing up in my urine back then.

I was beginning to wonder that, *at least in my case*, that the only tests that really mattered were the first and the last. The first one that diagnoses you with the mold infection; and the final one, where your mold toxins are at or near zero, and hopefully you're feeling good again.

Office Visit with a Liver Specialist on August 23, 2018:
After having a MRI on my liver in July, I met with my liver specialist Dr. J. In an earlier visit, he had declined to discuss with me a lab test from the Great Smokies Lab showing I had a damaged detox pathway in my liver. Apparently, if he was unfamiliar with the test, it wasn't important. In this visit, he said my liver was physically okay, and that my liver could not possibly be the cause of my pain in that area. When I asked him if my pain could be from a functional problem in my liver, he refused to consider it. He also dismissed the rash over my liver as a skin problem, not a liver problem.

Contact with a former Medical Doctor on August 25, 2018:
I had once seen Dr. C. as my primary care doctor when I had lived in Tucson, Arizona, in the early 2000s. When I looked her up on the Internet, I found that currently she was associated with the Arizona Center for Integrative Medicine at the University of Arizona.

In an email to Dr. C., I told her about Dr. Brewer's treatment for CFS and fibromyalgia. I knew that Tucson was a big area for fibromyalgia patients and for fibromyalgia studies. In her response, Dr. C. asked if I was seeing a functional medical doctor, which made me think maybe that was something I should look into.

<u>Office Visit with a Functional Medicine Doctor on September 20, 2018:</u>

I had a free consultation with this doctor, Dr. S., in Lawrence, Kansas.   He said he believed I was still going through benzodiazepine detox and withdrawal.

I told Dr. S. that I had a test from the Great Smokies Diagnostic Laboratory in Asheville, North Carolina, from back in 1997 called the *Functional Liver Detoxification Profile with Oxidative Stress Panel.* This test showed one of my liver detox pathways had shut down. My doctor, at that time, said this pathway that was shut down was the one that detoxes drugs from the body.

Dr. S. said that benzodiazepines like clonazepam get stored up in the tissues, and the drug needs to be detoxed out of the body after one stops taking it. That the benzodiazepines would get processed (metabolized) through the liver, and if my detox pathway was still damaged, this could be causing my liver pain.

The out-of-pocket cost of seeing Dr. S. on a regular basis was prohibitive for me; but for my benzodiazepine detox and withdrawal, he said he would recommend I read *The Ashton Manual* entitled *Benzodiazepines: How They Work And How To Withdraw*. See: https://www.benzo.org.uk/manual/contents.htm.

Dr. S. had also suggested I go on a detox diet plan under his guidance. However, from the materials he provided me, and from other materials I picked up on the Internet from the Institute of Functional Medicine, I began a semblance of this detox diet plan on my own. This was a dairy-free, whole grains only, and all organic (where possible) food diet.

For approximately the next two months of being on this diet, I slowly began to show some physical improvement in my physical strength and ability to function. After the first month, my liver pain faded. And by the week of November 18, I was having three or so good days a week, up from zero good days a week.

However, by the last week in November, I was very ill again. A sharp pain in my kidneys started then as well.

Also during this time, instead of my diarrhea improving, it became worse. But then I had read in *The Ashton Manual* that one of the problem areas with benzodiazepine withdrawal and detox could be gastrointestinal, including a problem such as diarrhea.

<u>Office Visit #27 with Dr. Brewer on December 3, 2018:</u>

In my notes for the doctor:

a. My continuing symptoms include sharp kidney pain, daily diarrhea, lessening liver pain, improving insomnia, and weakness and fatigue.

b. I noted my information about my August 23 visit with Dr. J., as well the information on my September 20 visit with the functional medicine doctor. I also listed what had happened with the mostly organic detox diet I'd been on.

c. I noted my recent stool testing by my new gastroenterologist was negative, and he recommended I have a colonoscopy and an endoscopy.

Dr. Brewer: "So this detox diet, you did it for one month, or are you still on it?" Bob: "I'm still on it. I started it [in late September]." Dr. Brewer: "And it is dairy-free, whole grains only, and all organic food?" Bob: "Not everything's organic, but most of it, as much as possible." Dr. Brewer: "And it seemed to help for three weeks?" Bob: "It helped up until last week. I seemed to be getting better every week until last week. Then I really had a bad week. But the week before that was pretty good."

We then went on to discuss my benzodiazepine withdrawal, which Dr. Brewer didn't believe was a factor any more. This was followed by a lengthy discussion about my health, and what had occurred and when. Most of the discussion focused on my long-term liver pain and diarrhea, but there was also some discussion on my more recent kidney pain.

Then Dr. Brewer said: "One of the other things that had occurred last fall, in 2017, in addition to the diarrhea and liver pain, there was a rash." … Bob: "Yes, I had a rash over my liver.

Somebody's looked at it and says it's not there. It looks like it's there to me, but it's so faded. It's something I've had ever since I had the CFS, off and on." Dr. Brewer: "You seemed to indicate it was new." … Bob: "The intensity was new."

Note: In Tucson, Arizona, I had an office visit in June 2003 with Dr. C. During this visit — after seeing a large, red rash over my liver — the doctor consulted several medical and alternative medical practitioners to try and determine what it was that she was seeing. Basically, what she came up with, *as I understood it,* was (a) the liver becomes damaged or impaired, causing sluggish functioning; (b) this creates excessive toxicity trying to get through the liver; and (c) having nowhere else to go, this excess toxicity comes out of the side of my liver, and then out through my skin, which is the cause of my skin discoloration over my liver area. I have often referred to this skin discoloration as a *rash.* ~~

Dr. Brewer: "First of all, I'll just talk about the mold briefly, then I'll kind of put it off to the side. Your tests were elevated back in June. Although it's pretty hard how to tie this all in with mold, I've had a few confusing cases lately. For example, I had a patient in six or eight weeks ago, whose mold test [numbers] were as high or higher than yours. And he feels fine. Best he's felt in years. So, go figure.

"In your test back in June, we were still showing quite a few mold toxins coming out of your body … [but] it's hard to relate mold to this whole story, with the liver pain, and the kidney pain, and the diarrhea, and all that. It doesn't seem to fit in. So at the moment, I think we ought to put it on the back burner."

After some more discussion on my liver, kidneys, and diarrhea, Dr. Brewer said: "The problem with CFS patients is, there is so much going on … The thing with you is, it did seem … you had done pretty well over the summer of '17 up through the fall of '17. And it does seem, that when you went off — and we must keep in mind it wasn't just one drug; it was also amitriptyline, you went off amitriptyline and clonazepam — everything went haywire the next day, and hasn't really been quite right since then." Dr. Brewer concluded by saying, basically, it was hard to understand what was going on with me.

<u>Chapter Seven: MCAS</u>

(A continuation of my office visit #27 on December 3, 2018)

<u>Mast Cell Activation Syndrome:</u>
Dr. Brewer: "Now I'm going to switch gears for a moment, because I don't think, in the last visit or two, have we talked at all about the mast cell activation?" Bob: "No." Dr. Brewer: "So we're going to switch gears, and this is going to be a whole new subject, and you've got new homework today. So it's like being in school, you've got new homework, because I know you like to get on the computer. …

"So the new thing I've been working on for about a year now — it's been kind of slow and methodical — is this thing called Mast Cell Activation Syndrome [MCAS]. It's kind of interesting how I got into this.

"About a year ago a patient gave me a book about MCAS. The book is written by a physician; he's an expert in it, and it's a pretty technically written book. The author, as I understand it, was writing it more for the general public, but it's written a lot more on the level of a physician. So my patient tried to read the book; it was way too complicated for them, and they gave up on it. And they brought the book in and gave it to me. I, obviously, breezed right through it.

"So I thought the book was absolutely fascinating, and shocking how much it fit with the majority of my patients in some way, shape, or another. So over the last year, I have been studying this a great deal. Not only did I read the book, I've read probably a 100 papers on it in the literature. I continue to read on it. I've talked to other physicians about it; and I've queried probably 200 to 400 patients of mine about it, about whether or not it may play [inaudible].

"It is interesting, the subtitle of the book. The book's called *Never Bet Against Occam: Mast Cell Activation Disease and the Modern Epidemics of Chronic Illness and Medical Complexity* by Lawrence Afrin, M.D. The subtitle of the book was, basically, that mast cell activation is responsible for the epidemic of chronic illness. The author comes right out and says he thinks it's the basis behind CFS and fibromyalgia, etc. He doesn't say in the book, but I think you could lump in chronic Lyme, EBV, and others in there. The beauty, as you'll understand in a moment, the beauty of the mast cell activation thing is that it would really explain a lot of things. It would explain many, many different things all ending up with the same set of symptoms.

"So what are mast cells? Mast cells are part of your immune system. They're basically a type of white blood cell. But they're also a very unique type of white blood cell.

"Most of the white blood cells circulate in the circulation; and then, if there's an infection someplace — be it in your kidney, your toe, your hand, or wherever — the white blood cells will move out of the circulation and go find the infection.

"So the mast cells are already out in the tissues. They don't reside in the blood stream. And they're everywhere in your body; every single square inch of your body; every organ in your body. Every place in your body has mast cells present.

"So the mast cells' role is to be the first alarm that sounds, the first warning to go off, when there's a threat to the body. When the mast cell activates, the mast cell will produce these chemical mediators, as they call them. These are a variety of chemicals; mast cells can make over 200 different chemicals, and then these are signals to other cells. Now the main cells that get signaled — not the only ones, but the main cells that are on the receiving end of these signals — are the rest of your immune system. So the mast cells are sort of the maestro for the orchestra of the rest of the immune system, but the orchestra can't start playing until the mast cell activates.

"So the main thing that will turn on a mast cell, not the only thing, as you will hear in a moment, but the main thing that will turn on a mast cell is an infection. Any infection. Could be EBV; could be HHV-6; it could be influenza; could be Lyme disease; it could be a staph infection; a urinary tract infection; anything. Any infection will turn on the mast cells. So after the mast cells activate, it produces these mediators — which includes cytokines, and histamines, and all these other things — and then those will activate the immune system to go fight the battle. In the scenario of an infection, once the battle has been fought, the mast cell quiets down; the immune system quiets down; everything goes back into a resting state, and you wait for the next problem to come along.

"So again, these mediators that are produced, these are like chemical emails to other cells, or signals to other cells, and there's a bunch of them. Some of the more common ones are again things like cytokines, histamine, etc. that will trigger these other cells. Histamine is a big one because mast cells are the major cell in the body that produces histamine.

"Now there's other things that can trigger mast cells above and beyond infection. A second one that's quite common, we are finding in our patients, are allergens. Mold could even come into that part of the equation. Mold, dust mites, pollens, ragweed, etc. What we're finding is a lot of our patients have long-standing allergies. Interestingly, some of our patients have had allergies all of their life. Some of them even have asthma. And then others, it's been more since they became ill. Either when they got Lyme disease, or EBV, or whatever, that seems to be when their allergies kicked in. I've seen both facets of it. But allergies do tie in with this.

"Now kind of in the same vein as allergies, this is probably the basis of chemical sensitivity, because as you may well know, a lot of CFS patients are chemical sensitive. And this is probably on the basis of mast cell activation, because a lot of chemicals will activate mast cells just like allergens will.

"Now the last one that's kind of interesting is that stress will activate mast cells. The stress can be subdivided into two kinds of stress: physical stress and emotional stress. Emotional stress speaks for itself, some very stressful emotional events in the person's life. Physical stress is a massively long list, of course. It could be trauma, surgery, even having a bad infection, etc. Could we throw benzodiazepine/amitriptyline withdrawal into that category? Maybe. Maybe taking those away on October 9, 2017, stressed your body enough that it sent you into a major mast cell activation. Maybe.

"What I've just described is, at least the part on infections and stress and so forth, is normal mast cell activation. We all have it. We all have trillions of mast cells inside of our body, and we probably wouldn't be alive without them, because again they're the first warning to go off to signal the onset of an infection, etc.

"MCAS, when you put that syndrome on it, is a different category. This is a group of patients in which their mast cells are not normal; they're abnormal. And they're abnormal in such a way that they activate too easily. They fire off too easily. What I mean by 'they fire off' is they release these mediators, these chemical emails, way too easily.

"Remember, I said before, let's say you get an infection someplace; the mast cells activate; they send signals to your immune system; the rest of your immune system activates; it goes and fights the battle; takes care of the infection, and everything quiets back down. The mast cells and the other white cells all go back into a normal resting state.

"With MCAS, that doesn't happen. The mast cells keep firing off, keep triggering inflammation. So the mast cells are way too twitchy, way too hyperactive; they release the mediators too easily, and it gets into a vicious cycle.

"So let's say that you have mast cell activation and I don't. Which, by the way, is probably the case. Because I'm certain I don't have it. I'm perfectly healthy. I'm not that much younger than you are. So let's say you have it and I don't. Why? Why do you have it and I don't? It's thought to be genetic. It's thought to be inherited.

"Data from Europe, over about the last couple of years, has suggested that this inherited MCAS afflicts about 15% to 20% of the population. So it's about one in five, one in six people. And again, it's inherited. Now most of my patients that we've gone into some detail discussing all of this can actually come up with family members that fit this.

"So the list of symptoms of MCAS is the longest list I've ever seen. It dwarfs CFS and Lyme and the others, but it includes all of those features. So it includes fatigue. The number one symptom by frequency of occurrence with MCAS is fatigue. It is the number one symptom. So if you took a thousand MCAS cases that were documented, fatigue would be their number one symptom. Other common ones are body pains like fibromyalgia, migraine headaches, IBS, asthma, allergies, anxiety, depression, rashes, etc. Sound familiar?" Bob: "Yes."

Then the doctor once again talked about how, if you're genetically predisposed to MCAS, there are a great many triggers that can set off the mast cells, including: infections, allergies, and stressful events.

"So let me give you an example. Let's take EBV. So you've got two teenage girls, different families, that are in seventh grade, and they both get mono the same day. And one of them genetically has MCAS and the other one does not. The one without the MCAS gets a little sick with the mono; misses about a week of school; is fine a couple of weeks later, and is back to normal life. And she never has any problems the rest of her life. The one that did have MCAS becomes chronically ill; can't get the mono whipped, and has this chronic inflammation/CFS issue that goes on the rest of their life. And I have patients like that, and it did start with documented mono. I have probably 50 patients like that.

"So, 80% to 90% of the whole general population has had mono. Why do only a certain subset get sick? Now I'm not sure I'm right on that, but I think it makes a whole lot of sense. So that's exactly what I'm saying. In a genetically predisposed person, you set off this vicious cycle of inflammation and it's hard to get under control.

"The other issue with MCAS is, it's not always the same thing that sets it off. So years ago in you, it could have been

EBV. If EBV goes active, it can keep setting it off. At another time, it could have been allergies. At another time, it could have been stress. At another time, it could have been something else.

"So it's curious to wonder — on October 10, 2017 — if your body just said, 'Uh-uh, we're not going to do this, fellow. You're not going to get by without clonazepam and amitriptyline. We're not going to make this easy on you.' And it was stressful to your body, and it could have set it off. That's conjecture, but it sort of fits.

"And I'll tell you, Robert, the more I get into this, I'm telling you one of the most common symptoms I see with this is irritable bowel syndrome [IBS]. I bet I see 10 cases a month of patients when we get into a discussion about their bowels. With you, it's new. You never had it before November 2017.

"So as I've gotten into this, I've also seen some very interesting cases. Now let me tell you about this one interesting lady I saw. I've been seeing her for about a year. It's a fascinating story. So this gal, in retrospect, if you go through her history, she fits exactly with MCAS. She had allergies as a kid; she's had allergies all of her life; and she's prone to getting skin rashes, like hives and so forth. She had a few migraines, which goes along with MCAS. But she basically led a pretty normal life. I mean, she was fine; she worked out; had a good job, and everything was basically fine."

Bob: "You can have this syndrome and not know it until it gets triggered?"

Dr. Brewer: "Correct. I call [the triggering events] nuclear bombs. So she was basically fine, for the most part, until March 2017. In March 2017, she develops a sudden GI infection. Now we don't even know what it was, because she never went to the doctor. She just assumed she would get over it. So she got fever to about 103, and had about 15 watery bowel movements a day. The severe part of it lasted about three days. … If you give me one guess, I'd probably say it was norovirus. But we don't know what it was. … And then the fever went away, and the diarrhea went from about 15 to 20 watery bowel movements a day down to about six to eight.

"But then she absolutely fell off a cliff. By 'fall off a cliff' I mean she then developed chronic — which she has to this day, I just saw her about a month ago — she has chronic abdominal and bowel problems. So now we're almost two years [later]. So she has abdominal pain; diarrhea, which is not as bad now as it used to be; bloating; etc. So she has all these abdominal problems that never got better after that, but she has profound CFS.

"When I first met her, she only left her house to go to doctors' appointments. Fatigue, migraine headaches, aching all over her body, fibromyalgia-like aching, lightheadedness, numbness and tingling, and it just went on and on. She felt like she was dying. And again, the whole thing started with some kind of a GI infection in March 2017. She can tell you the day and the time. …

"And again, when you talk to her, her background history … She's got a whole family, like her sister has Lupus, and she's got another sister with fibromyalgia. And so the family tree fits. And I've got several other interesting cases like that. But hers is very interesting in that it started with a GI problem. And one of her major symptoms that's still going on is diarrhea. Not as bad as it used to be, but it is diarrhea.

"Unfortunately, the testing for MCAS is not well-covered by insurance. It's very esoteric testing, so usually it's just a clinical diagnosis. But there is one thing we can do with you. Give me your pen and paper. [I complied.] Roll up your sleeve. [I did.]

"You're going to be positive. I'm going to mark on your arm, but I'm not going to use ink. I'm just going to kind of scratch your arm, a little bit like a scratch test. You can watch. I'm just going to draw an 'X' there. [This he did, but he didn't press overly hard; and he used the tip of my pen to do it, but with the point retracted; and he did it on the inside part of my lower right arm.] We're going to see if that turns pink and red. It's already starting to turn. So we'll watch this here for a minute or two.

"This is called dermatographism. 'Dermato' means skin; 'graphism' means writing. Writing on the skin. But again, we're not using ink. So yours is going to be pretty dramatically abnormal. You can already see the 'X.' See it?" Bob: "Yes." Dr. Brewer: "In a lot of people, this really starts to burn." Bob: "And I'm color blind." The doctor laughed.

Dr. Brewer: "In a lot of people, this really starts to burn, and itch too. I had one young man that we did this on, and he said, 'Oh, this is going to be a problem.' And I said, 'What do you mean?' And he said, 'Watch.' And … it marched up his entire arm and turned red all the way across the chest. Within minutes. So that's pretty abnormal.

"So this doesn't happen in me at all. You can draw on me all day long and this will not happen. I've done it to myself. So in the general population, this only occurs in about 5% of people. So it's abnormal. That's in a general, healthy population. See, I'm in the 95%. I don't do dermatographism at all. It doesn't affect me at all. … [But with my patients] I probably haven't seen a normal one in three to four months. I'll see maybe one normal one out of 50 to 100 patients."

Bob: "But this 'X' indicates I have the syndrome?" Dr. Brewer: "This indicates you have the syndrome. Because what's happening is, you've got thousands of mast cells under your skin, and … just the downward pressure of an object — like the blunt tip of my pen, but you could use a stick or anything, tip of a spoon, you can use anything — the downward pressure of the object on the skin leads to histamine release from the mast cells. Which they should not be doing that, just a little downward pressure on the skin should not do that. So it means your mast cells are way too twitchy; they activate too easily, and just the pressure releases it. This is pretty much 100% histamine, what we just did. That's why it can itch and burn.

"I've had one patient in — swear to God, these are true stories — I've had one patient [where the] mark on their skin lasted for a week. And I've had another patient [where the mark] lasted a month. …

"So [the 'X' on your arm] strongly indicates you probably have it. And what do we do about it? We try to minimize the triggers. Like, in your case, anything you're allergic to, try to avoid, like mold. And that's why, if we think — if mold, EBV, whatever is a trigger— we try to keep those minimized.

"I've been playing around quite a bit — it's still kind of in its infancy stages — but I've been playing around quite a bit with antihistamines and things like that, to see if they'll help. And that comes right out of the book. The guy in the book writes a lot about various things to try, like antihistamines. Like Claritin, Zyrtec, and that sort of thing. So there may be a variety of things to try."

Bob: "So when I was exposed to the mold in the flood waters where I lived, and I was sick for six months with flu-like symptoms, that triggered the syndrome, and that brought on the full …" Dr. Brewer: "Yes. Absolutely. That's the thing. There can be multiple different triggers. It's like, mold was probably a huge problem back then, but it may not be now. And I still can't explain why your [mycotoxin] levels are so high, but you're not the only one."

Bob: "You said you store these toxins up in your tissues, and then you detox them." Dr. Brewer: "You do. At least these ones we can measure; we can't measure the benzodiazepines. We can measure these. Maybe this functional doctor's right, but we can't measure them. We don't have any blood tests to measure benzodiazepine." Bob: "I joined this Facebook group, but I haven't read it yet. It's all for people on benzodiazepine withdrawal. I'm going to see what people write."

Dr. Brewer: "It is interesting. The guy that wrote the book, one of the things that he sometimes uses to treat MCAS is — this is quite interesting — so one of the things he uses to treat it is benzodiazepines, because benzodiazepines will quiet down mast cells. So I wonder if the benzodiazepines were keeping them kind of quiet, and when you took the benzodiazepine away, the mast cells said, 'No, no, no. You can't get away with that.'" Bob: "Wow." Dr. Brewer: "Isn't that interesting?" Bob: "Yes."

Dr. Brewer: "Off the top of my head, I can't remember if he used any amitriptyline for treatment. He's written a lot on treatment, the guy that wrote the book. You could try to work your way through the book. The doctor's name is Dr. Afrin. The book is really tough to get through, for the average person. But I tell people, if they've got a lot of spare time, if they want to wade through it, it's in paperback.

"But I think you probably have it. I think there have been a number of different triggers over the years. You wonder if something had to have happened on October 10, 2017. And the problem is, now you've got this whole GI thing going on. I think, 'Okay, so what should we do at this point?'"

I mentioned my nurse practitioner was going to refer me to a nephrologist, and that perhaps I should see a kidney doctor before I did any colonoscopy and endoscopy testing.

Dr. Brewer: "I don't mind you seeing a kidney specialist, that's fine. It's probably not a bad idea. I think they'll find that your kidneys are going to be okay." Bob: "That's what I would think too. They've been tested before, and they couldn't find anything." Dr. Brewer: "Right. The GI thing, because diarrhea is new — it's not new-new; you've had it for about a year — I do think you probably should proceed with the colonoscopy and endoscopy, just to make sure they don't find any colitis. I'll have an occasional person come along, that have had CFS for years, and all of a sudden, 'Bam,' they've got ulcerative colitis.

"By the way, this MCAS they think ties in with autoimmune disease. So lupus, Crohn's, ulcerative colitis, Hashimoto's thyroiditis, rheumatoid arthritis, MS, etc. Even psoriasis. So it's thought this may be the basis of autoimmune. You can almost see when the mast cells go nuts. And they set off this vicious cycle, and you start making autoantibodies."

Bob: "Do you think the PEA that you talked about would help with this?" Dr. Brewer: "Oh, I think it's great. I hear good stuff about it all day long." Bob: "I did try the PEA. I didn't notice anything from it, but I still have some left. I can try that again." Dr. Brewer: "Yes, I'm using it on everybody. Now I will say, I've had some patients who didn't notice much change. I've had other patients just absolutely adore it. They love it."

We discussed when we had talked about the PEA before in regards to my fatty liver. Dr. Brewer: "Yes. I think you should get back on it." Bob: "Do you have any idea about dose?" Dr. Brewer: "One twice a day. … I think, after you get the GI workup done, and if it's clear. Because I don't want to start you on anything until we know that you don't have colitis, or something like that. So I do like the idea of getting the GI workup completed.

"Now the one GI doc had talked about putting you back on amitriptyline, but you never did do that. Is that correct?" Bob: "I went back on it for a while, but it didn't seem to do anything at all. I was like on it for three months on a real low dose, so I stopped it." Dr. Brewer: "I'm actually glad you did that, because it would suggest that — because remember, you stopped them both at the same time on October 9, 2017 — so it would suggest that it was actually the benzodiazepines that set you off. Or the benzodiazepine withdrawal."

Bob: "So if I have this GI workup, I should let you know?" Dr. Brewer: "Yes, because I've kind of got a protocol that I'm working on. PEA's on there. I kind of got a protocol of things. One of the things — and again, this is not me, it came right out of the book — one of the things I start with is antihistamines. Claritin, Zyrtec, that sort of thing. And then we work up from there. …

Bob: "Since I appear to have this syndrome, that could be behind my problems?" Dr. Brewer: "All of it. From a genetic standpoint, right. Yes, it could be behind everything."

Bob: "And how does this fit in? I mean, if someone [doesn't] have the mold. I have a friend with Bartonella, could this be …" Dr. Brewer: "Oh, absolutely.   Any infection, any allergy. Bartonella will do it." Bob: "So if someone had Bartonella and extreme chemical sensitivity, would they be a candidate for some kind of protocol like this?" Dr. Brewer: "Yes. It's all MCAS. I think you all have it. That's my opinion." …

Bob: "So people you're treating for mold, and they still have the CFS, do you do mast cell stuff at the same time?" Dr. Brewer: "Yes." Bob: "So you've added this in with your CFS protocol?" Dr. Brewer: "Yes, yes. For sure."

Two Books on MCAS and CFS Reviewed:

(1) *Never Bet Against Occam: Mast Cell Activation Disease and the Modern Epidemics of Chronic Illness and Medical Complexity* (2016) by Dr. Lawrence B. Afrin.

Following my December 2018 office visit with Dr. Brewer, I bought and read this paperback book. In it, the author talked about *mast cell activation syndrome* (MCAS). The author also referred to MCAS as *mast cell disease.*

Dr. Afrin said MCAS was seen as a more frequent form of mastocytosis. Mastocytosis itself is a rare form of mast cell activation disease (MCAD) that has been medically recognized since the late 1800s.

The doctor/author wrote that, besides improper mast cell activation, there was also improper mast cell mediator production and release. In seeing his early MCAS patients, overall Dr. Afrin believed that the release of these mast cell mediators could be seen in a wide variety of patterns, which then led to the large range of symptoms that he saw in his patients. In this, the doctor found it hard to fathom a disease more complex than this mast cell activation disease.

Dr. Afrin went on in his book to describe some generalities and some of the major issues that were seen in MCAS.

<u>A statement made by Dr. Afrin that was of special note to me:</u>
He said that weight gain in MCAS patients, even as much as 100 pounds, were common; and that this could happen even when there was no change in eating habits and physical activity.

This very thing happened to me back in the early 2000s, when I was not doing too badly with my health, and when I was on a diet and steadily losing weight. One morning I got up and weighed myself, and I saw I had gained three pounds. I thought it must have been an anomaly. But the same thing happened again the next day. And the next. This went on for more than two weeks. I was freaked-out by it, and I began to wonder if the weight increases would ever stop. But then they did stop, just as suddenly as they had started. Perhaps one or more of the homeopathic remedies and/or herbal tinctures I was taking at the time turned out to be a mast cell stabilizer.

<u>Another statement of special note to me:</u>
Dr. Afrin wrote that MCAS may cause inflammation and pain in the liver.

<u>More on the book:</u>
Dr. Afrin did talk about a lack of diagnostic criteria for MCAS. With this being the case, Dr. Afrin emphasized the importance of ruling out potential alternative diagnoses.

Treatment for MCAS was discussed from pages 216 to 234. Dr. Afrin started out by listing some general principles in the treatment of MCAS before getting into the treatment options for the illness.

In concluding his information on treating MCAS, Dr. Afrin stressed the importance of finding a local physician that would partner with you to help you successfully manage the chronic issues seen in MCAS.

Diagnosis of MCAS (chapter 26); understanding the unknowns in the illness (chapter 27), and effective medical care (chapter 28), are all things the doctor said may remain elusive for some years to come.

<u>The Treatment for MCAS:</u>

I used Dr. Afrin's *Treatment for MCAS* section of the book as a jumping off place for gathering information about treating MCAS, getting the same as well as additional information from off the Internet.

First, however, I would like to mention some of Dr. Brewer's additional comments from two emails I got from him in early February 2019:

a. Dr. Brewer said that he had seen a number of patients who were very sensitive to medications and supplements. He said he had communicated with Dr. Afrin about this, and Dr. Afrin felt that most of these sensitivities arose from the excipients or fillers used in these products. For instance, Dr. Brewer said he had seen several patients who were reactive to the *quercetin*, one of the main supplements used in treating MCAS.

b. Dr. Brewer does not prescribe benzodiazepines for his MCAS patients. He feels "there is too much down side with dependence, etc." However, he did say that he would reserve its use "for severe, unrelenting cases."

c. Dr. Brewer said that, in keeping with what Dr. Afrin had said, he has "had the most success with antihistamines so far" in treating MCAS. When I asked what antihistamine was reported to be working the best, he said the OTC antihistamines. He followed that up by saying he usually starts the patient off with "generic Claritin, at one pill once or twice a day."

<u>The Treatment Options:</u>

<u>Antihistamines:</u> there are both histamine 1 and histamine 2 receptor blockers:

a. Histamine 1 receptor blockers include: Claritin, Alavert, Allegra, Zyrtec, Xyzal, and Atarax. This list also included Doxepin, a tricyclic antidepressant.

b. OTC Histamine 2 antihistamines can help with gastrointestinal symptoms and overall mast cell stability. These are basically antacids: prescription Axid, and the OTC drugs Pepcid and Tagamet.

<u>Ketotifen:</u> It is said to be a mast cell stabilizer, and it's available only through a doctor's prescription. I don't know how readily available the ketotifen is, but I've read that some patients have purchased ketotifen capsules through compounding pharmacies.

<u>Some Supplements:</u>

a. Stinging Nettle: there are four parts — roots, stems, leaves, and flowers. The leaves and stems are an antihistamine.

b. Butter bur: is an antihistamine.

c. Mangosteen: is an antihistamine and an anti-inflammatory.

d. Ginger: a mast cell stabilizer, antihistamine, and an anti-inflammatory.

e. Bromelain: an enzyme found only in pineapple juice and in the pineapple stem. It's a mast cell stabilizer, an anti-inflammatory, and an antihistamine.

<u>Warning:</u> The next section deals with the essential oils. Unless you are experienced in their use, I would advise against using essential oils except under the guidance of an experienced health care practitioner. Otherwise, questions will arise with their use: am I allergic or reactive to an oil; which oil do I use for which problem; do I use an oil full strength or diluted in a carrier oil; etc.? Also, what quality of oil do you buy: 100% pure; organic; unprocessed with chemicals; etc.? ~~

<u>Some Essential Oils:</u>
a. Peppermint oil is said to be the safest of the oils to use in MCAS because it has a low potential for triggering mast cell activity. It is also said to be an antihistamine and a mast cell stabilizer.
b. Ginger has mast cell stabilizing properties.
c. Rosemary, fennel, German chamomile, and thyme help detox the liver. All four oils contain flavonoids, and fennel and German chamomile are also anti-inflammatories.
d. Orange is a strong anti-inflammatory, a pain reducer, and it contains flavonoids that inhibit mast cell activity.
e. Juniper berry is high in flavonoids; it helps detox the liver, and it supports liver function.

f. Holy basil contains two flavonoids; is a mast cell stabilizer, and it alleviates inflammation and eases pain.

g. Lavender inhibits mast cell activity.

h. Turmeric contains flavonoids, and it is also an anti-inflammatory and an antioxidant.

i. Celery seed contains flavonoids, and it is also a detox aid and an anti-inflammatory.

j. Yuzu contains four flavonoids.

<u>NSAIDs:</u> "These are anti-inflammatory drugs that reduce pain, fever, and inflammation. Such drugs may be helpful in MCAS, but Dr. Afrin warns that they may also trigger flares in MCAS patients. NSAIDs include aspirin and ibuprofen (Advil, Motrin).

<u>Opioids:</u> In general, opioids stir up mast cells in MCAS and cause the release of histamine. However, *tramadol* appears to be the exception, and it is the only opioid acceptable for use in mast cell disease.

<u>Flavonoids:</u> The flavonoids have antihistamine and anti-inflammatory properties, and there are four kinds:

a. Quercetin is the *master flavonoid,* and it is one of the best of the natural antihistamines.

b. Green tea extract inhibits mast cell activation; it has the flavonoid catechin in it.

c. Citrus bioflavonoids found in citrus fruits.

   d. Grape seed extract and Pycnogenol.

<u>Other:</u>
a. Resveratrol: is considered to be a mast cell stabilizer.
b. Blueberries: are said to be a natural mast cell regulator.

<u>Benzodiazepines:</u> includes Ativan, clonazepam (the generic form of Klonopin), Xanax, and Valium.

<u>Cromolyn:</u> is a drug obtained from a compounding pharmacy, and it is known to be a mast cell stabilizer and an anti-inflammatory.

<u>Other Supplements:</u> These may be of help, as either natural antihistamines and/or as mast cell stabilizers:
a. alpha lipoic acid and N-acetylcysteine (NAC)
b. ascorbic acid (vitamin C)
c. DAO (diamine oxidase enzymes)
d. omega-3 fatty acids

This list of helpful items to take in treating mast cell disease is by no means all-inclusive. Also, more items in this area can be found in Dr. Afrin's book.

(2) *Toxic: Heal Your Body from Mold Toxicity, Lyme Disease, Multiple Chemical Sensitivities, and Chronic Environmental Illness* (2018) by Neil Nathan, MD.

I found this book addressed many of the issues that I had and that no one else ever seemed to talk about.

In my reading, Dr. Nathan started out by addressing the problems of what he called his *ultra-sensitive patients.* These patients were sensitive to, and had a hyperactive response to, a great many things — such as drugs, supplements, etc.

He also discussed his patients who had problems with excess toxicity, where the patient's organs of elimination didn't or couldn't do their job.

Thus many of Dr. Nathan's patients were both sensitive and toxic. He had found that many things, such as homeopathic remedies, might help these patients.

Dr. Nathan mentioned that doing a detox protocol might be best for many patients as the first step of their treatment. He even mentioned some products he had found to be helpful in this area.

Then Dr. Nathan went on to write about mold and its treatment, mentioning both Dr. Ritchie Shoemaker's and Dr. Brewer's treatment protocols.

Next he discussed Bartonella infection and its treatment.

Then Dr. Nathan's book included a chapter entitled *Mast Cell Activation Syndrome.* He said that, besides the toxic mold issues seen in CFS, mast cell disease was another big player in the chronic illness of many of the patients he sees. Dr. Nathan went on to discuss mast cell illness, including treatment for MCAS. He did mention that mold toxicity was the most common trigger for MCAS; and that when you treat the trigger successfully, the MCAS often disappears.

The rest of Dr. Nathan's book went on to discuss many more areas of interest.

This is a good book, in my opinion, for any CFS, fibromyalgia, and Lyme disease patient to read — especially ones who are very chemically sensitive and/or who have detox problems. For several years I had been looking for just such a book, with this kind of information included in it, before finding and reading this book of Dr. Nathan's.

Office Visit #28 with Dr. Brewer June 4, 2019:

In my notes for the doctor:

(1) My main complaint remains the sharp pain in my liver. I know the doctor said at our last meeting that my liver pain could be from the liver, but that it also could be from something else, and that we didn't have the lab work to show what the problem was exactly. I want to speak to this:

a. In March 1995, I had the *Functional Liver Detoxification Profile with Oxidative Stress Panel* test done by the Great Smokies Diagnostic Laboratory in Asheville, North Carolina. The doctor that ordered this test was CFS specialist Dr. Scott Rigden, who back then was practicing in Tempe, Arizona. The liver (and gut) problems in CFS at the time were his area of medical research. Dr. Rigden said my lab test was substantially abnormal and that it showed that one of the detoxification pathways in my liver had shut down. Two other CFS specialists, Dr. Eileen Wright of Orlando and Dr. Evan Kligman of Tucson, who were both familiar with this lab test, at later dates told me that they supported Dr. Rigden's findings.

b. For over 20 years, when I have had pain in my liver area, I have taken either milk thistle or phosphatidyl choline to aid in liver functioning. Both supplements are well-known liver aids, and both have relieved my liver pain over the past 20 plus years up until October 2017. While this may not be conclusive proof of it, I believe it's highly probable that the pain in my liver area is actual liver pain. In any event, this colors the way I view my current liver issues.

Note: Dr. Rigden wrote an article about his research and treatment of liver and gut issues in CFS. It was entitled *Entero-Hepatic Resuscitation Program for CFIDS*, and it was published in The CFIDS Chronicle, volume 8, No. 2, Spring 1995, pages 46 through 49. (CFIDS is another name for CFS, and it stands for Chronic Fatigue and Immune Dysfunction Syndrome.)

Dr. Rigden believed that many of the symptoms associated with CFIDS/CFS were associated with chronic toxicity, and that this could be caused by poorly functioning detoxification organs, specifically the liver and the gut; and that this in turn could lead to a damaging accumulation of toxins in the body.

(This sounded similar to some of what I read in Dr. Nathan's book, and similar to Dr. Cheney calling CFS [in part] a *toxicity disorder* back in 1999.)

I don't know how many CFS patients may have one or both of the liver and gut problems Dr. Rigden described. All Dr. Rigden wrote in this area was that, in his study of 200 CFIDS patients, 80% of them indicated the capacity for clinical improvement with his entero-hepatic resuscitation treatment. ~~

(2) Events since my last visit:

a. Mid-December 2018: I read Dr. Afrin's book and want to note that he said that MCAS might cause liver pain and inflammation. (See p. 132 in his book.)

b. I tried several supplements, some of which Dr. Afrin had mentioned in his book, that are supposed to be helpful with MCAS. These were (at one capsule/tablet a day, but which I had an adverse reaction to): vitamin C (1,000 mg); PEA; the flavonoid supplements quercetin, rutin, luteolin, and those in green tea; NAC and R-lipoic Acid; generic Claritin (loratadine); generic Pepcid (famotidine), and blueberry. Finally, 500 mg of the vitamin C again (but only once every three days).

c. Since my last visit on February 19, 2019: I went on a prescribed dose of 10 mg of Doxepin for depression and anxiety, but I've read the drug is also supposed to be good for mast cell disease. By prescription, I later upped that dose in March to 20 mg daily.

d. March 12: I went on the prescription opioid tramadol for extreme liver pain. I started out by taking 75 mg of the drug twice daily.

e. March 27: Since I'd had problems with taking flavonoids and other supplements for my MCAS, I went searching for something new that might help with my liver pain. It was then that I came up with the essential oil holy basil, heavily diluted, for application over my liver. This essential oil is said to alleviate inflammation and ease pain, and it contains two flavonoids which have shown the ability to stabilize mast cell activity. The holy basil oil has since proven to be helpful in controlling my liver pain.

f. April 20: I dropped the holy basil oil and added-in German chamomile essential oil, heavily diluted in a carrier oil, for application over my liver. This essential oil is said to contain 36 flavonoids; it stimulates the liver; it's helpful to the liver in releasing toxins, and it is an anti-inflammatory and an antihistamine. It has also been helpful in controlling my liver pain.

g. Early May: I thought that if detox stirs up the liver mast cells and they produce my liver pain, helping the liver detox and controlling mast cell activity during these times might help alleviate that pain — even to the point of getting off the tramadol. Also, since January, I've read Dr. Nathan's book *Toxic*. I identified with some of the patients that he wrote about. That is, I am sensitive to treatment therapies, and I have a problem with detox. To this end, through an acquaintance, I obtained two tinctures from Beyond Balance, the company I wanted Dr. Brewer to sign up with as a practitioner. (These were products used by Dr. Nathan.)

h. May 11: I started taking the Beyond Balance tincture product called Tox-Ease GL, one drop in water, at 1:15 a.m. In Traditional Chinese Medicine, the liver is most active from 1 to 3 a.m. My liver pain is at its worst at 3 a.m., and it's the only time the essential oils don't fully help with the liver pain. My experience with adding in the Tox-Ease GL has been that, for the first time, the tramadol has almost fully controlled my 3 a.m. liver pain.

i. May 15: Also at 1:15 a.m., I dropped the German chamomile oil and added-in orange essential oil that is said to suppress mast cell activity. My experience with adding-in the orange oil was that my sleep afterwards was longer and deeper, and my overall liver pain decreased even more.

After the doctor reviewed my file and my visit notes, we briefly discussed my liver situation.

Q. What little research information I could find suggests that toxicity may be the underlying cause of the mast cell disturbance in the liver. This may be true. When I first tried the German chamomile essential oil (heavily diluted) over my liver, I soon noticed I had a detox reaction in my liver. My liver pain also increased substantially. Based on this, it appeared to me it was possible that my liver detox problem aggravated my now active mast cells in my liver, which in turn aggravated my liver pain. Did the doctor have a comment on this?

A. "So you're saying the chamomile helped, but before it helped, you had these worsening symptoms?" Bob: "Yes." Dr. Brewer: "How long did that last?" Me: "Just a day." Dr. Brewer: "Oh, just a day. That hasn't recurred?" Me: "No. But I had the same thing with the orange oil that I tried. It's like a detox reaction."

Dr. Brewer: "I think you're right. I think that's a reasonable assumption." He said when the toxins are "embedded inside of a cell or a tissue, the mast cells can't see the toxins. … [But when the toxins] come out of the tissues, the mast cells can see them. … [And then the] mast cells will react to the toxins. … So yes, I think that's a reasonable assumption. It's kind of like a Herxheimer reaction."

Q. Since I keep having these UTI infections — indeed, I've read UTI infections are common is MCAS — what does the doctor think about my taking supplements to prevent more UTIs? I'm already on cranberry and probiotics, but I've read D-mannose can be good for this recurring problem.

A. "As supplements go for UTIs, that's the two that I've heard. Cranberry we actually use a lot of. Cranberry extract. A lot of patients use that, particularly women, for UTIs. And I've also heard that D-mannose works."

Q. Later this month, I plan to add-in the Beyond Balance tincture called Mast-Ease to help with overall control of my mast cell disease. (I have tried the Mast-Ease, and while I was not reactive to it, it was too much to use at the same time as when I was starting out using the essential oils.) As we previously discussed, if I need more of the Beyond Balance products, I would appreciate it if the doctor would then sign up as a practitioner on the Beyond Balance website at: https://beyondbalanceinc.com.

A. We discussed my use of the Beyond Balance products, the Tox-Ease GL (a tincture to assist with liver detox) and the Mast-Ease (a tincture to help control mast cell activity). When I need more of the Beyond Balance products, the doctor said to let him know by email and he would then sign up as a practitioner for me, so I will be able to order them directly instead of through a third party.

Q. Could some sort of overall MCAS treatment help with my liver pain, as well as help me feel better overall? Besides my wanting to try the Mast-Ease that Dr. Nathan uses, is Dr. Brewer seeing anything new that is helping his patients with their MCAS? Are there any compounding pharmacies out there that are compounding small doses of some of the flavonoids, with no problematic excipients or fillers?

A. "You are correct in that Dr. Afrin feels that, in a lot of these medications and supplements, that the excipients are a big issue with mast cell patients. ...

"Now compounding pharmacies can try and make medications without excipients, but I don't know about supplements. You'd have to call someplace like — you've got King [pharmacy] over in Lawrence — you'd just have to call one of them and ask them." Bob: "I found one that was totally 100% organic, with no excipients, and the fillers were supposed to be non-problematic. But that's the only one I found. It was just a supplement over the counter."

Dr. Brewer: "Right. And that's your best chance, to just keep digging online and look for ones that don't have any additives, excipients, and fillers. Those are thought to be a problem. Afrin just says that over and over. It's no use to argue with him; he's seen over 3,000 mast cell cases now."

Q. With the essential oils and Tox-Ease GL, I am down to taking 75 mg of the tramadol once a day for my liver pain. It's my hope that eventually I'll be able to use a high enough dose of these products to control my liver pain so that I won't need the tramadol any longer. I've read that the tramadol is the only opioid that doesn't aggravate MCAS. I also feel like it helps tamp down the MCAS — is that possible? And what should I be on guard about when using an opioid like the tramadol?

A. "So with the Tox-Ease, you're down to taking 75 mg of Tramadol. What was your amount before?" Bob: "75 mg twice a day. Now I'm down to once a day. I'm actually surprised that the oils have worked as well as they did."

Dr. Brewer: "I am too, Robert. I'm really surprised. I mean, I've had lots of people who have tried essential oils for Lyme and mold and things, and some of them topically. They rub them on their feet, hands, and arms. You may be the first one that's rubbed it on your liver, on the abdomen over the liver, but I'm surprised they've worked as well as they have." Bob: "They were 100% organic too. That might have been helpful."

Dr. Brewer: "I don't know about the tramadol. I think your first part is correct, it's not supposed to aggravate mast cells. I don't know if it tamps it down or not, but that is interesting. I don't know." Bob: "It seemed to, but I didn't know for sure. I wasn't positive about it."

Dr. Brewer: "It's kind of in that same vein, as there's so many things that come up. ... I belong to a mast cell doctors' discussion group now, that I joined in about December. And so I get probably — that's part of how all my emails get buried — because I get about 20, 25 emails a day from them. But the doctors will bring up these interesting patients, and all kinds of weird stuff they see and say. Does anybody think this could be part of mast cell activation? And almost everything that comes up — of course Dr. Afrin is the main person; he's the one that started the group, and he usually gives a lot of the responses — but almost everything that comes up somehow ties-in with mast cell activation."

Bob: "In that book of his, there are so many symptoms." ... Dr. Brewer: "It's incredible. Hundreds. I had one patient who read the book, and was only half way through, and listed her own personal symptoms that she had found in the book, and she had about 40. … Now she's very ill. She's got a lot of issues."

Q. I find I am more debilitated and more ill with the MCAS than I was with the CFS/mold (except when I had to go into hospice care with the CFS/heart problem). I also have some symptoms that come and then completely go, like depression and anxiety. Is the doctor seeing these same things with many of his other patients?

A. "The answer is 'yes,' although a number of mast cell patients are improving. They're feeling better. With some of the things you've tried and can't take. Like the Claritin, and PEA, and so forth."

Bob: "The point of taking the one drop of the Mast-Ease is to eventually build up to five or six drops. Then to eventually build up so that I can take a supplement every three or four days. That's my goal." Dr. Brewer: "The Mast-Ease, I assume from the name, is directed at mast cells. Correct?" Bob: "Yes. In Dr. Nathan's book, those are two he recommended. The Tox-Ease for liver detox, and the Mast-Ease for mast cells."

Q. I have read that MCAS can lead to disease progression in the liver, including with fatty liver. I have also read that disease progression with fatty liver, at its worst, is cirrhosis and liver failure. According to Dr. J., my fatty liver hasn't changed from my liver biopsy in 2006 to my MRI in 2018. So, should I be worried about my fatty liver and the apparent MCAS activity in my liver?

A. "So this question about fatty liver is all correct. Mast cells probably can enhance fatty liver, and you should be worried. Now I wouldn't set around and stew about it all day long, but yes, your liver must be monitored. I mean, just because we've diagnosed you with that, it doesn't mean anything's been changed for the worse, other than you found you react to a whole lot of stuff. But yes, you need to keep an eye on your liver. Through the medical profession, I mean. What you've heard from Dr. J. is good news, but everything you've said in here is correct."

Q. After I wrote the previous question, my latest CAT scan results (May 2019) came in showing my fatty liver had actually *improved*. Could this be from my diet — which is fish and fowl (red meat and pork-free), gluten-free, dairy-free, low salt, low sugar, and 100% organic whenever possible?

A. "It showed improvement?" Bob: "Yes, that's what they said." Dr. Brewer: "Wow. I mean, that's great." Bob: "Yes. Everybody was shocked. I didn't know ..." Dr. Brewer: "It could be dietary, but it also could be some of these things you're taking. Some of these oils and stuff. And maybe the Beyond Balance.

"One thing I was going to mention, which might be in some of the stuff you take, not in the oils, is ... One of my patients brought in an article for me a few weeks ago on berberine. Which is an herb; it's basically goldenseal. And this specific article was on fatty liver. They had shown berberine had helped fatty liver. But that might be in some of your stuff, I don't know. I'd have to look at the whole list." Bob: "Would that be worthwhile taking? It's a supplement?" Dr. Brewer: "Yes. But cross-check it with the Mast-Ease, because maybe it's already in there. As you know, it's a pretty common herb."

Q. Did the doctor's patients who relapsed after their successful mold treatment relapse because the mold returned, or because they had active MCAS, or both? **A.** "So your question about relapsing after successful treatment of mold, I think it's some of each. Some people, the mold returns. And in some of them, it's the MCAS. I think it's some of both."

Bob: "I feel like I'm on the right track, as far as I've gotten, anyway." Dr. Brewer: "Yes. I wish it were some other way. You hear from all these other mast cell doctors, there's a whole lot of trial and error. And you've been through it. And unfortunately, so much of it is these darned excipients and fillers. And additives." Bob: "Yes, I wondered, because I shouldn't have had such a bad reaction to vitamin C." Dr. Brewer: "Yes. We've heard from other patients.

"So the three oils you mentioned, you're still using all three?" Bob: "Yes." Dr. Brewer: "And you're using the Tox-Ease? You do have some Mast-Ease, but you haven't …" Bob: "Yes, I have the Mast-Ease. I tried it for a couple of days, and I felt it was too much with the oils I was starting on. So I have a bottle of that." Dr. Brewer: "Right. You're planning on restarting it?" Bob: "Yes." Dr. Brewer: "Small dose?" Bob: "One drop a day, probably." Dr. Brewer: "On the Tox-Ease, are you still using one drop?" Bob: "Yes. On the Tox-Ease I'm still using one drop. I'm surprised I actually felt something from using one drop. But I'm pretty sensitive." Dr. Brewer: "I would think that is a very accurate statement. You are very sensitive, but you're not alone."

Then Dr. Brewer said: "I think I have something in here, from your last visit, you had had some diarrhea last go-round. Is that settled down now?" Bob: "With the tramadol, I find I get constipated. Then I have to take a laxative or a stool softener, and then I'll have a normal bowel movement, and then I'll have some diarrhea afterwards." Dr. Brewer: "You wouldn't think your baseline bowel pattern would be diarrhea?" Bob: "No."

After a brief pause, Dr. Brewer said: "So, with your day-to-day routine these days … is fatigue still a big issue?" Bob: "Yes." Dr. Brewer: "There's a new supplement that has come out; I'll actually give you a handout on it. I don't know if you've ever gotten anything through Researched Nutritionals before; I suspect you have." Bob: "Yes." Dr. Brewer: "So you have an account there?" Bob: "Yes."

Dr. Brewer: "So it's called ATP 360. I think it just came out in April. I found out about it probably just before the 1st of May. There was a scientific conference down in Arizona in early May, largely about mold. It was not the only subject, but I would say about 60% of the talks were on mold, which I gave one. Dr. Nathan was one of the organizers of the conference, so I spent a couple of days with him. It was actually a very good conference."

Bob: "Are there videos on it? Available to the public?" Dr. Brewer: "I don't know. Write down 'ISEAI,' which stands for International Society for Environmentally Acquired Illness. That was the name of the conference. You can go to their website; it's something like https://iseai.org. They'll have them there if they have any that are available. [I did this later, and I couldn't find any such videos available.]

"Anyway, right before this conference, the Researched Nutritionals person was in and was telling me about this ATP 360. They had a booth at the conference, and they had a lot of information about it. It's basically, and it's kind of a cool idea, it's a lot of stuff you've taken before. I will caution, it does have vitamin C in it, but there's not very much. But it's got magnesium, riboflavin, CoQ10." Bob: "I've taken some kind of ATP, but it wasn't Researched Nutritionals." Dr. Brewer: "This one's new. This is a combination of about 12 different supplements, and it's for mitochondrial support. That's what it's designed for.

"The interesting part of it is, they've got [an eight week] study — which they'll have on their website — and they actually took patients with fatigue … and they put them on this ATP 360. And there was a 50% reduction in fatigue in eight weeks. That's a lot.

"So I've got probably somewhere around 10 patients who have started it. Because, remember, I just found out about it a month ago. But I haven't had any feedback yet. The person who's been on it the longest may have been on it two weeks, three weeks. I told people that, if they see something really positive, to call and let us know, so we'll be able to share that with other patients. But obviously it's way too early. Not even close to eight weeks yet. But you might be interested in it. You can find it on their website, but I'll give you a piece of paper on it. They have a flyer on it that I just made a copy of."

The doctor left and returned with a copy of the flyer.

Dr. Brewer: "One of the talks was on 'Cell Damage Repair' [CDR]. So there's a research group at the University of California at San Diego that has studied this whole CDR mechanism, and its all about mitochondrial damage from infections, toxins, etc. And … you have to get the cells and the mitochondria back to a healing phase, and back to normal, and in some patients, that's very hard to do. … It's kind of interesting; I heard about this about a week before the conference. Then we get this big talk on mitochondria.

"So anyway, you might be interested in trying [the ATP 360]. If you try it, start real slow. The dose on there is three capsules a day. Don't start with three. Just start with like one, or whatever. And you might want to wait until you're on the Mast-Ease. You might want to get it restarted first."

Bob: "And this cell damage repair thing is …" Dr. Brewer: "It's a theory. In other words, it's not some supplement or something. … They have a huge amount of research into it. It's pretty darn interesting." Bob: "So you're saying it's something I can go read?" Dr. Brewer: "Yes. It's on the Internet." Bob: "And I just look for cell damage repair?" Dr. Brewer: "And the main researcher, he was the guy who gave the talk, his name is [Robert] Naviaux. A really cool guy. Just phenomenal. I think he's actually got some YouTube videos on the Internet. There's quite a bit of free stuff on the Internet. I just looked it up the other day.

"It's kind of a whole new … The thing is, it ties in with CFS, and Lyme, and mold toxins, and everything, even mast cell activation — all these things that create inflammation or toxicity. It even ties in with slow detoxing, because if you have too much toxic effect hanging around with your cells, it's going to damage them and damage the mitochondria."

Bob: "So does he talk about how to repair that damage?" Dr. Brewer: "Yes. He thinks this kind of stuff helps. They've got kind of an experimental thing they're working on, which is on some of this YouTube stuff. It's not available, but they're looking at all kinds of different options. At the moment he has more of the model that looks to be correct, from a cellular standpoint. But not the exact fix. But he does say this stuff helps. Not specifically this one, but mitochondrial support supplements."

We ended the visit by discussing the ingredients in the ATP 360, which I could read off the flyer he had given me on the supplement.

<u>Request of the Doctor on September 17, 2019:</u>
I asked Dr. Brewer for a Cromolyn prescription. I also asked that the prescription come with [a sucrose filler], keeping my MCAS in mind. (The pharmacy offered to use any of about eight different fillers.) The doctor replied the following day: "Will order 200 mg size capsules which is the standard size. People usually need 200 mg 4X per day to respond, but OK to start slow. Ordered #90 with refills."

The doctor did order the Cromolyn, at a cost of $88, from the CareFirst Specialty Pharmacy that I had found online at: https://www.cfspharmacy.pharmacy.

<u>FaceTime Visit #29 with Dr. Brewer on May 21, 2020:</u>

In my notes for the doctor:
a. From June 4, 2019, until mid-September: in an attempt to control my mast cell disease and its associated problems, I

tried various items such as nettle leaf and ginger root (that was said to contain no fillers and excipients). My body couldn't handle them. I had more success with the many oils I tried: rosemary and yuzu (liver); sandalwood, vanilla, lily, and tulip (sleep); and cypress (anxiety and depression). [For anxiety and depression, my nurse practitioner had tried increasing the Doxepin I was on from 20 mg to 25 mg daily, but it had proved too high a dosage for me to handle.]

b. After having several UTI infections last summer through the fall, I saw a urologist. In a CAT scan he ordered, it showed I had bladder stones. I underwent surgery December 27 to remove the stones, and to have a surgical procedure to help me empty my bladder more fully (which I was told would help keep me from developing bladder stones again.) I got another UTI while I was still in the hospital, and another UTI in mid-January 2020. My surgeon said this was not uncommon with the surgery I'd had.   On February 7, after completing two more rounds of antibiotics (from year-end and mid-January), I felt much better.

c. February 14: I noticed the very sharp, early morning liver pain had eased back down to a mild liver pain, which seemingly meant the mast cell activity in my liver had slowed. I tapered off and then stopped the tramadol I'd been on for over a year. Now my nurse practitioner says my liver enzymes are the best she's ever seen them (since I went on the essential oils for the MCAS liver activity).

d. This spring, since having surgery for bladder stones, I have been struggling a lot with (1) lack of energy, (2) mild liver pain, (3) mild kidney pain, (4) soft or watery stools, and (5) shortness of breath.   After 27 years of CFS, I strongly suspect some of this is a detox problem. I also know my liver has felt sluggish lately, and that's been part of the problem. A few weeks back I started using, over my liver, the essential oils of turmeric (an anti-inflammatory, antioxidant, with some flavonoids), and celery seed (a detox aid, an anti-inflammatory, with some flavonoids). [I used both oils heavily diluted in an almond carrier oil.] This has since somewhat helped improve my energy levels and overall health.

I went over for the doctor my information on the several UTIs I'd had in mid-to-late 2019, and the surgery I'd had to remove my bladder stones at year-end 2019. (My UTIs and my surgery were why I had missed my December visit with the doctor.)

Dr. Brewer: "Obviously you've had a real mess with these UTIs, which part of that was the bladder stones. ... The tie in with the mast cell activation is, any kind of an infection can kick up the mast cells. ... And then they're slow to calm back down. So with these recurrent UTIs you had, dating clear back to last fall, I think that kept you kicked up and inflamed a lot of the time. The question is, are [the UTIs] gone, or are they going to start kicking up again. … Obviously the surgery was hard on you." Bob: "Very hard."

Dr. Brewer: "The liver pain I've never completely understood with you. Is it due to the fatty liver? But yet, I think you've been told in the past your fatty liver isn't that bad, right?" Bob: "Yes. And it hasn't changed since …" Dr. Brewer: "It hasn't changed any on the scans, so …" Bob: "Yes, 15 years, so …"

Dr. Brewer: "So your liver pain I don't understand. I don't know why. And I don't know why it cranks up at a certain time of day. It's weird. Maybe you're on to something with the detox, but I don't know." Bob: "I had this test, years ago, that showed one of my detox pathways was damaged. So I don't detox well. And you and I talked — it's been a year, and maybe it's longer since we talked about this specifically — but we talked about how, if I'm struggling with detox, that's kicking up the MCAS in my liver, and that could be generating pain." Dr. Brewer: "Right. And I think that's still plausible."

Bob: "And I think that's why the oils with the flavonoids in them, put over the liver, have helped with the pain. Because it's come down, and I've been able to get off the tramadol." Dr. Brewer: "Right. You just put those [essential oils] on your skin, right?" Bob: "Yes."

Q. In my notes for this office visit, I asked about all the antibiotics I'd been on, and the UTIs I'd had, and the effect they could have had on my MCAS.

A. "Unfortunately, the problem with the mast cell activation is that there can be so many things coming at you from different directions. Not getting proper sleep stresses your body, which probably kicks up mast cells. The UTIs kick up mast cells. If you're right about the detox thing in your liver, that may kick up mast cells. So you always have multiple factors coming in at once. But I tell people, you just have to tackle them individually and try to get them under the best control possible. ... You've at least gotten the stones out of your bladder and had the surgery, so maybe the UTIs will calm down. You've done a good job in attacking the things that we know about, and you're doing some things that may be helping with the detoxing of your liver."

Q. Does anyone know what causes the extreme fatigue in mast cell disease? **A.** "No, [but] presumably [it's] because the mast cells produce a lot of those cytokines and so forth that produce the flu-like phenomenon. [With] mono, flu, any kind of infection like that, fatigue is a common symptom. It's probably, in the broad term, inflammation that's giving rise to the fatigue as well as the other symptoms."

I noted that, from mid-September to mid-October last year, I had experimented a little with taking the Researched Nutritionals supplement ATP 360, and then the drug Cromolyn. At that time, they proved too strong for my body to handle.

Note: In the discussion that follows, the dosage of the ATP 360 I was taking was a half a capsule every three days, and the recommended dosage was three capsules daily. ~~

Dr. Brewer: "So tell me how you did the Cromolyn. How much did you take?" Bob: "25 mg." Dr. Brewer: "So one fourth of an ampule?" Bob: "Yes." Dr. Brewer: "Once a day?" Bob: "Every three days." Dr. Brewer: "Oh, wow." Bob: "It just kind of kicked my butt. It might have been because I was having the UTIs and on the antibiotics. It might not have just been a good time when I tried it."

Dr. Brewer: "Yes. The mast cell experts say that about half, or maybe more, of the patients show good responses to Cromolyn. Some get side effects, so that's why they recommend go low, start slow. Take it very slow, which obviously you took it extraordinarily slow.

"I did talk to a patient earlier this week who is a CFS patient with mast cell. He went slow, but not nearly as slow as you. He did 100 mg once a day, one ampule once a day, for two to three weeks, and then he just kept slowly increasing it. He's now up to four ampules a day, and it's the best he's felt in 25 years. He basically said it's nothing short of a miracle.

"Some of the other stuff has worked with him, the antihistamines and some stuff like that, but he said the Cromolyn's been incredible. But that may not apply to everybody. I'm trying more and more of it. I don't have a lot of feedback yet, but I do have a number of patients who are doing quite well on it. I think it would be worth a try again. Gosh, starting at that low of a dose shouldn't bother you."

Bob: "I started to raise it, because I felt a little better, a kind of a little buzz when I started it. And then, when I increased it, I didn't feel so good. But I had a lot of UTI stuff going on, and the antibiotics, so ..." Dr. Brewer: "Yes, those UTIs are a mess because ... I'm telling you, with those, you were not rid of those, Robert. While the stones were there, you had constant infections, because the bacteria grow right on the stones and you can't get them off of there. You had continuous UTI, even though you may not have felt it all the time. You had continuous UTI because it grows right on the stones.

"When you increased the Cromolyn, what did you do? Did you just go more frequent, or a higher dose?" Bob: "A higher dose." Dr. Brewer: "Like a half?" Bob: "Yes." Dr. Brewer: "How long did you wait to increase it?" Bob: "A week."

Dr. Brewer: "So this guy says — the guy I talked to the other day, he's done quite a bit of research on the internet about Cromolyn — and he said a lot of sites on the Internet say it takes two to six weeks for it to stabilize its effect. So he would say a week is too fast. He went every two to three weeks. Now he did start at a higher dose, a 100 [mg dose] daily, one ampule daily, but he went every two to three weeks. So it took him several months to get up to four a day.

"So I think it's fine to start back at that low dose, but I would not increase it for at least two weeks."

We discussed the prescription I had, and at one point Dr. Brewer asked: "It's a liquid that's in there, right?" Bob: "No. It's a powder." Thinking it was in liquid form, that could have been why the doctor was talking about ampules instead of capsules. And I have only seen people on my mast cell disease discussion list mention ampules, not capsules.

Dr. Brewer: "So I would take it slowly, but don't increase it until you feel like … If it's not bothering you at all, or you're getting a little better, then you can increase it. And I'd make that at least a minimum of two weeks. And like I said, I learned that trick this week from the patient who's doing so well on it. I think it's worth trying again. Now do not do the ATP 360 at the same time. Do one at a time, because [if not], you know what happens. You start mixing and matching, and then you don't know what's going on."

Q. My primary care doctor did say recently my thyroid indicated I needed to be on thyroid medication, which he then went ahead and prescribed for me. It's Levothyroxine, at a dose of 25 mcg to start with. I'm not sure when to take it, because taking it when it's time for most people to get up for the day is not workable for me. I'm usually taking supplements for my liver and kidneys then, which helps calm my organs for sleeping. So, does it matter when I take that? **A.** "It does, but of course you're not on a usual schedule." He said this because of my awful sleeping hours, grabbing sleep when I could throughout each 24 hour period, which meant my sleep times varied from day-to-day.

Bob: "Just as long as I take it at the same time everyday, and some period of time with no food before and after?" Dr. Brewer: "I think so."

We then discussed how I had been on it years ago, when I had first gotten sick, but not since then.

Dr. Brewer: "That's another one I hear a lot about, is thyroid. This is about the fifth time I've talked about it in a patient this week. It's a common thing we hear, is the thyroid situation. And it can be tricky to get it regulated. And with thyroid, you need to go slow. I'm sure your doctor told you that. Usually they start — and that is a low dose — they usually start with a low dose and work it up slowly.

"See … we think thyroid plays in with mast cells. … There's some people that think that mast cell activation actually leads to the thyroid problems; but then, if the thyroid's out of whack, it activates the mast cells. So again, another vicious cycle. But you're addressing it, so that's good.

Q. At this point in time, does the doctor have any thoughts on whether his patients will be able to take the Coronavirus vaccine when one becomes available? **A.** "A lot of mast cell patients react to vaccines. … I mean, if a person's taken other vaccines in the past — like the flu vaccine, the pneumonia vaccine, stuff like that — and they did not react, they'll probably be alright."

Dr. Brewer: "You've got to stay on top of this UTI thing. Let's hope and pray that getting rid of those bladder stones has taken care of it, and now your bladder's emptying better. Let's hope that takes care of it, because I'm telling you, any time you have infections going like that, it's just going to throw you completely out of whack."

Then the doctor went back and briefly touched on all the other things I needed to stay on top of, including: taking the Cromolyn again; he's fine with my use of the essential oils; taking the thyroid medication. He said: "You're doing all the right things."

I asked, "So you're saying definitely, like if I experience more UTIs, or more extreme kidney pain, I should go back to the urologist and stay on top of that?" He said: "Yes. Yes. Right."

Q. I'm still seeing articles on CFS speculating as to causation, such as it being caused by the thyroid, etc. Also, that I had kept a running commentary on my treatment for mold etc. since June 2013. This included my notes, as well as [partial] written transcriptions of the audio recordings of my office visits with the doctor. So, if my health allowed, I was thinking of putting this information out in a self-published, 125 (?) page booklet on https://www.amazon.com (except the cost would probably be prohibitive). Or perhaps putting it out on Facebook, or on some other website, or offering the information free on a website that had discussions on CFS. What does Dr. Brewer think of this? I'm not sure what I think of the idea myself, but at least two CFS patients I've shared my summary with said they had found it helpful. They have also said they thought it was a good presentation. **A.** "I think it's fascinating. I think it's kind of a cool idea."

We then discussed the options for putting this out there and the possible prohibitive cost. He said, outside of self-publishing on Amazon, "I would explore your other online avenues, like Facebook."

After a bit more discussion, the doctor said, "I kind of like the idea. I mean, you obviously study this; you have collected a lot of information over the years, so…"

I then told the doctor about my friend Steve who had been a CFS patient in a Sacramento nursing home. After I sent him Dr. Brewer's information, Steve had found a doctor to treat him with Dr. Brewer's protocols. Steve was now completely recovered, and he was back to living on his own again in his own apartment.

Dr. Brewer: "And that was mold, right?" Bob: "Yes. He had lived in a trailer for a while, and he later discovered it was full of mold." Dr. Brewer: "I have quite a few patients for whom mold has been the key. I think mold is very common in a lot of CFS cases — as we showed in our papers and so forth — but in some of them, it is a deep, deep problem. With others, like you, it's a mixed bag.   But in some of them, [mold] is the primary problem."

We hadn't discussed one of my questions at this point, so I brought it up before our visit concluded. Bob: "When I first got that mast cell activation, I was sicker and more disabled than I was with [just] the CFS. But since I've had the UTIs and the surgery, I don't feel as bad now as I did then. You think that the antibiotics, or the surgery, or all those infections, could have somehow changed that activity?"

Dr. Brewer: "I do. … I'm telling you, with the constant UTI, the mast cells are just firing off all the time. I do think that's what happened. I think it's a combination of all those. The antibiotics helped keep the infections down, but couldn't get rid of them until you did the surgery to get rid of the bladder stones. … So I agree with you, the mast cells may have calmed down because they're not being triggered. Because with mast cells, it's all about triggers. So at least, as best we can tell, the UTI triggers are calming down now."

<u>HHV-6 Reactivation:</u>

June 7, 2020: I believed my latent HHV-6 virus had reactivated. Also, if this was similar to what had happened with me back in 2016, the HHV-6 reactivation would soon be accompanied by an EBV reactivation. The way I had begun feeling was quite a bit different from the way I had felt in the past with the MCAS, and it was very reminiscent of the way I had felt before when the HHV-6/EBV viruses had reactivated. Because of this, I started back on an old prescription I had of the valacyclovir, and I would eventually add-in the transfer factor PlasMyc.

Email to Dr. Brewer on July 6, 2020:

I sent Dr. Brewer an email detailing the above, and I asked him for a new prescription for the valacyclovir. I also asked:

a.   Could I still be detoxing mold toxins out of my body; and if so, could that have led to my reactivated HHV-6/EBV activity?

b.   Should I do another mold test from RealTime Labs?

Dr. Brewer responded that same day: "I will send in a new Rx for valacyclovir - 1 gram, #90, of which you can continue to take 1/2 twice daily. I will order another mold test (urine kit) and we can mail it. Dr. B."

Letter from Dr. Brewer dated August 14, 2020:

Dr. Brewer wrote: "I have received back your urine mycotoxin assay results (copy enclosed). You do have modest elevation of aflatoxin and gliotoxin (both produced by Aspergillus). It is tough to know if this is contributing to your symptoms or not, but it is certainly possible. I do not recall if you are still using the nasal spray or not. Let me know where you are at with the nasal spray, and then we can come up with some ideas. I assume that there are no obvious mold issues in your apartment."

I went ahead and reviewed the enclosed mycotoxin test results from RealTime Labs dated August 11, 2020. I would put my thoughts on these lab results in my notes for the doctor that I wanted to discuss at our next office visit.

Still, it was apparent to me that the higher levels of the mold toxins yet to be detoxed out of my tissues were continuing to suppress my immune system. This would have allowed any reactivated HHV-6/EBV infections to occur.

Blood Draw on August 17, 2020:

As part of this lab work — which was ordered by my primary care doctor — I asked the local walk-in clinic doing the blood draw to also run lab tests to determine if I had possible active EBV and HHV-6 infections. After all my lab test results were back on September 2, the next day I faxed them to Dr. Brewer.

In a cover letter that went along with the faxed test results, I asked if "either or both these [herpes virus] tests show active infections?" I explained that "the walk-in clinic nurse practitioner [who had done the blood draw] said the EBV test only showed past infection [which I thought was incorrect]; and that the HHV-6 test showed I was a 'carrier' [whatever that meant]." I also explained that my regular primary care doctor said he didn't know how to read these tests.

<u>Email from Dr. Brewer on September 4, 2020:</u>

Dr. Brewer said he was responding to my HHV-6/EBV test results, and my questions about them, by letter. He also attached "a very interesting recent paper on HHV-6/CFS/mitochondria. It is technical but you will get the overview: basically, partial reactivation of HHV-6 impairs the mitochondria."

The article also said that the impaired mitochondria led to lower cellular ATP and a lowered immune system response.

<u>Letter from Dr. Brewer received on September 11, 2020:</u>

I received a letter (dated September 4) from Dr. Brewer. In it, he said:

"The HHV-6 (type B) is too high. As you can see, you have 18,000 copies, and it should be less than 1,000."

[According to my research on the Internet, a virus' DNA particles are called *copies*. These copies are reported per milliliter of a blood sample, such as in *copies/mL*. A high number of copies indicate a rapid viral replication; a low number of copies indicate an inactive infection.]

"I would probably favor you going on the transfer factor Multi-Immune. This is the transfer factor that has immune boosting capabilities. This may help down-regulate 'partial reactivation' of the HHV-6. I suppose we could try valacyclovir, although there is not much data that it helps with HHV-6 (as opposed to EBV where it may be somewhat helpful). I think the best shot is trying to improve your immune system, including the natural killer cell function."

First, I wondered why the doctor had said "partial reactivation of the HHV-6" instead of activated HHV-6. Also, this same term was used in the medical article he had sent me September 4 in an email attachment. I made a note to ask the doctor about the meaning of this terminology at our next office visit in November.

Second, I thought the transfer factor mentioned might help my friend Steve in California with his near non-existent natural killer cell count, so I emailed him the information.

Otherwise, I was perplexed by Dr. Brewer's response in that he did not review my EBV test. I made a note to ask him about that EBV test result at my next office visit.

FaceTime Visit #30 with Dr. Brewer on November 17, 2020:
Note: At this point I had been on my gluten-free, dairy-free, mostly organic diet for some time. Then, about four weeks before this office visit, I changed my daily diet by cutting out chips (tortilla and potato); popcorn cooked in oil, and non-dairy, *nut* milk frozen desserts. The effect of this seemed to be a lessening of my liver pain. Then two days before this office visit, I again changed my diet by cutting out nuts (except pecans) and cooking oils (except sesame seed oil). Within 24 hours, my health was surprisingly much improved. I didn't feel sickly at all, and I was much stronger. ~~

In my notes for the doctor:

a. I became very ill soon after our last visit. It felt a lot different from the mast cell activity of 2019. I thought it was because my HHV-6 had reactivated.

b. June 7: I started back on an old prescription of valacyclovir, at one half of a one gram tablet taken twice daily. (I updated to a new prescription of the valacyclovir from the doctor July 7.)

c. June 28: After 21 days, I cut back the valacyclovir to one half of a one gram tablet daily, and for the first time I added one half of a capsule of the PlasMyc transfer factor.

d. July 24: After a total of 47 days, I went on a maintenance dose of half a capsule of the PlasMyc twice daily and stopped the valacyclovir. (I was on the valacyclovir/ PlasMyc for approximately 46 days in late 2016, and then again in early 2017, and that had proved effective back then.)

e. August 20: After another 27 days, I cut my maintenance dose of half a capsule of the PlasMyc to once a day.

My current Symptoms: I'm feeling like I'm knocked out all the time (fatigue, weakness); and I have watery stools, and liver and kidney pain. It doesn't feel like herpes viruses or MCAS now, but more like some kind of prolonged die-off.

To begin our visit, I verified for Dr. Brewer I was still on the PlasMyc at half a capsule once a day.

Bob: "I was talking to a friend of mine this weekend, and I couldn't understand why I kept feeling so bad, and she suggested it could be my liver. So we went over my diet and changed a couple of things, and I started feeling better; and feeling better, I feel like I need to be back on the valacyclovir.

Dr. Brewer: "Yes. So your symptoms [that have] persisted for these last several months have been fatigue and weakness, and then you've had the kidney pain?" Bob: "Yes. And the liver pain." Dr. Brewer: "Those are the biggies?" Bob: "Yes. The kidney pain seemed to get better when I did two things. I was on the PlasMyc and valacyclovir, but also that August 17 lab testing showed I was slightly dehydrated, so I've been drinking a lot more water. So the pain has gone way down on the kidneys, and I don't know whether it's because of the antivirals, or water, or both. I would guess both." …

Q. Part A: Per my August 17 blood work, did I actually test positive for active EBV?

— and —

Q. Part B: While talking with another CFS patient, the idea came up that maybe I'd been having a low-level HHV-6 infection for some time. I didn't know if this was possible, so I looked it up. According to HHV-6 Foundation website, a person can have a "low-grade acute infection" or a "low-level persistent infection." And this low-level infection doesn't show up on most HHV-6 testing. Then the doctor sent me an article, attached to an email, which the doctor said was "a very interesting recent paper on HHV-6/CFS/mitochondria." Basically, that paper said partial reactivation of HHV-6 impairs the mitochondria.

a. Does the term "partial reactivation of HHV-6" in the article mean the same thing as a HHV-6 "low-grade acute infection" or a HHV-6 "low-level persistent infection" that I have wondered about?

b. Is there a difference health-wise in a fully-blown HHV-6 infection and a partial reactivation of HHV-6?

c. Wouldn't an HHV-6 partial activation make it easier for HHV-6 and EBV viruses to fully reactivate?

d. Wouldn't an HHV-6 partial activation, along with the mold toxins suppression of the immune system, indicate the need to be taking a maintenance dose of the valacyclovir/PlasMyc until all the mold toxins have been detoxed out of the body?

e. If I had a HHV-6 partial activation, could this aggravate other health conditions?

Note: The article/paper referred to in our discussion is entitled: "Human Herpesvirus-6 Reactivation, Mitochondrial Fragmentation, and the Coordination of Antiviral and Metabolic Phenotypes in Myalgic Encephalomyelitis/Chronic Fatigue Syndrome," and it can be seen at: https://pubmed.ncbi.nlm.nih.gov/32327453/. ~~

A: "So, probably the hardest of your questions — not your fault, it's the nature of the beast — the hardest ones we deal with are these darn HHV-6 and EBV issues.   Just as a sidelight, you probably heard that Covid patients are now, some of them, are evolving into CFS." Bob: "Yes, I heard that the other day." Dr. Brewer: "And it's a pretty large number of them.   I mean, of course there are so many people that have had it, millions have had it. So this shows how these viruses can set off a sequence of events, and then continue to cause persistent symptoms afterward.

"Now the difference is, the Covid virus actually does eventually go away, out of the nose and lungs and so forth, whereas ones like EBV and HHV-6 hang around forever, at least in a dormant form.   So there's still — and you're a prime example of this — an ongoing issue of how active is this HHV-6, EBV, or both?   And then, to what degree are they playing with your symptoms?

"Now the blood work that you've had done, the HHV-6 — you've had this at least twice now, and I'm including that one that wasn't too long ago — the HHV-6 is actually the DNA in the virus. I mean, when they do that HHV-6 PCR test on your blood, that's the actual virus DNA. So that's not supposed to be there. You're not supposed to have HHV-6 virus floating around in your blood. So that would suggest that it's active.

"The EBV, we have a DNA test for that, and I don't know that you've ever had that done."   Bob: "It was in that blood work from August 17." Dr. Brewer: "Yes, but that's antibody testing. At any rate, we've had a couple of blood tests on you, over the last three years, that have shown HHV-6 in your blood. The actual virus.

"And then, I don't know that we've actually ever done … There is a test for the actual virus on EBV, but we rarely find positives.   But then we sometimes think it's active if the antibodies are elevated, which then gets us to the August 17 blood work — now this is for the EBV we're talking about at the moment — and it's kind of 'maybe.'x

"Now the other problem is, which antivirals will work on those? Let me go into a little bit of this question [on the] partial reactivation [of the HHV-6] that came out of that mitochondrial paper that I told you about last time. What they say in that paper is — and again, all this terminology came out of that paper; not all of it, but the term *partial reactivation* came out of that paper — and what they said in there is, there is not active virus. There is not full reproducing virus, so it is not producing new virus particles. But it's making some of the early proteins that the virus would use to assemble a fully active virus, should it go that far, but it doesn't go that far. Now we have no idea what that means.

"This is all new research about this whole partial reactivation. They suggest that, in some shape or form, the partial reactivation may screw up the mitochondria, which are responsible for energy production.   And I haven't really heard anything new on that subject since that paper was published.

"Now when we get into like low-grade activation and that sort of thing, we're talking about actual live, reproducing virus. So the HHV-6 test that you had, I think twice now over the last three years or so, showed the HHV-6 DNA in your blood. That's actual reproducing virus. So that would be, at least a low amount of active …

"Because, see, with the partial reactivation, it's really like the virus is inactive, but it's starting to turn on about 20%, but that doesn't actually produce a live virus particle. But what we find in your blood, with HHV-6, is actually live virus particles." Bob: "Is it only the live virus particles that make you sick?"   Dr. Brewer: "We don't know.   That's the problem.   A lot of your questions are really good, but we don't know the answers.

"So the other question is, does the same thing occur with EBV, because they're cousin viruses? They both can produce a mono-like illness. So can the same thing occur with EBV? Now your EBV blood tests that were done on August 17, those are antibody tests. So those are your immune system reacting to the virus. But we've used those over the years, including in you, to try and get an idea if the virus might be active.   And your antibody tests are not as low as we would expect if you were a healthy person walking around on the street, but they're not sky high.   So I think the question of 'could the EBV be active?' is somewhere between 'maybe' and 'probably' on you.

"Now the other question is, treating these viruses. Valacyclovir, what you took back in June, probably works pretty well for EBV. I've had some — and it's not just me, other doctors around the country have done this for decades — I think valacyclovir can be effective for EBV. And I like your idea of going back on it. The problem is the HHV-6. It probably doesn't work very well for HHV-6. Now we don't know that a 100%, but at least, based on test tube studies and so forth, it's not very effective. Valganciclovir, Valcyte, which of course is a lot more expensive and so forth, it may be active against HHV-6.

"I saw an interesting Internet post on one of our infectious diseases' sites recently. Try this one on for size. This one's really wild, Robert. This one's crazy. So this infectious disease doctor, I can't remember what state he was from, took some of these still-sick Covid patients — not meaning sick from the respiratory Covid illness itself, but [sick with] fatigue, brain fog, achiness, etc.; a kind of a chronic fatigue-type illness that had developed in his Covid patients. And he found some laboratory evidence, a little bit different than what you had done, but he had some laboratory evidence of HHV-6. He treated them with valganciclovir and they improved. So could HHV-6 be reactivating in some of these Covid patients? Maybe."

Here we had some trouble with our FaceTime connection and we had to reestablish the call. However, we could only hear one another and not see each other except for a blurred screen. This used up a couple of minutes of our time.

Dr. Brewer: "So at any rate, there is some question of maybe HHV-6 playing a role in some of these Covid patients. That will be an interesting subject to follow. And the guy didn't say anything; the guy that put this post on our website didn't say anything about EBV, just HHV-6.

"So, to summarize, here's what I think we ought to do with you. I think you should go back on the valacyclovir. Take that for a while — taking it along with the PlasMyc is okay — and see how you do. See how you feel over the next couple two or three months. Then, if you're still struggling and not showing some improvement, then we should probably repeat that HHV-6 blood test. The one you've been positive for previously. Because the valacyclovir may not work for the HHV-6, and we need to see if that rascal is still around. Then we'd have to make a decision about valganciclovir. Does that sound reasonable?"

Bob: "Yes. Oh, I had something I thought about this morning. I remember in that letter you sent me, you talked about Research Nutritionals' Transfer Factor Multi-Immune. Can you take two transfer factors at the same time?" Dr. Brewer: "Yes, you can. Particularly when you're taking smaller doses, like you're taking a half capsule of the PlasMyc. Yes, you can."

Q. Kidney pain: My kidney pain goes back as far as 2011, when I had an ultrasound on my abdomen, and then a CAT scan on my abdomen in November 2019. According to the doctors ordering the tests, no problems were seen with my kidneys at either time.

Also, the doctor has said that the mycotoxins pass out of the body through your kidneys. From medical websites, I have read that mycotoxins can: harm kidney tissues, promote kidney toxicity, and do kidney damage. In addition, I have read EBV can cause kidney inflammation. This makes me wonder, can my kidney pain be due to continuing mycotoxin detox and low-level HHV-6 activity?

A: "You know, I've really never understood your kidney pain. Could HHV-6 or MCAS or whatever cause that? I don't know. I think inflammation in your body seems to be associated with it. I think you and I both agree on that. Because we know that people like you have inflammation, and we know that can be triggered by a variety of mechanisms like viruses, mold, mast cell activation, etc. I don't think it's from the mycotoxins. Didn't you tell me that with the valacyclovir, the PlasMyc, and then drinking more water after that, your kidney pain improved?" Bob: "Oh, yes. Dramatically. It's a lot better."

Q: Per my recent mycotoxin test with RealTime Labs: I tested negative for aflatoxin in 2013; my apartment tested negative for mold in 2013; I was then treated with nasal antifungals in 2013 and 2014, with dead mold coming out of my nostrils in late 2014. Regarding my latest mycotoxin test:

a. The ochratoxin is down from 2.8 in 2013 to now 1.43 (not present).

b. The trichothecene is down from .38 in 2013 to now .029 (equivocal).

c. The gliotoxin is down from 2.76 in 2016 to now 1.71 (present).

d. The aflatoxin has gone up from -0- in 2013/2015 to now 1.768 (present).

Note: *Present* meant at infection levels; *Equivocal* meant possible infection; *Not Present* meant no infection. ~~

Q. I believe that I'm still detoxing mycotoxins out of my tissues. If I see one of the first three mycotoxins reverse course and go back up, I will want to do the nasal antifungal again.

a. Has the doctor ever seen a mycotoxin level behave like my aflatoxin level? How could this happen?

b. Surely the mycotoxin levels present are suppressing my immune system?

c. Surely if I tried the far infrared sauna therapy at this point it would put too much pressure on my liver and kidneys?

A: "[Per your question on] your mold toxin test, that one's actually the easiest of all to answer. So here's the deal. … They changed the aflatoxin assay between the 2013, 2014 time range, and the current assay is much more sensitive. It picks up aflatoxins easier than the old assay. So you can't compare old results to new ones. I know they do on that little chart [on the bottom of the test results page], but that's not correct. Because we have patients that never, ever measured positive for aflatoxin, and now they've got tons of it. So the difference was the assay. See, your others went down, so it could be … I have a ton of people who were zero back in 2012, '13, '14. And now I rarely get a zero on aflatoxin. I used to. So I wouldn't worry about your aflatoxins.

"You know, you didn't look too bad. Your gliotoxins was 1.71; ochratoxin was 1.43. You still got a little bit of a low level, but they're not bad. I don't think we want to completely ignore them, but they've certainly improved over where they were in the past. And I think you had mentioned, I know it's hard to tell, but this doesn't really feel like mold toxicity to you, correct?" Bob: "Yes."

Q: I have a friend who got better after being on the nasal amphotericin for three years plus. And now, even though he's got his health back again, his natural killer cell levels remain at *one*. … Now that he's off the amphotericin, should the NK cells return to normal? Would the Researched Nutritionals transfer factor Multi-Immune help my friend with this NK cell issue?

A: Dr. Brewer: "You know, I'm still intrigued, after all these years, why the NK cells are low [in CFS patients]. Is that a viral mechanism? Is it mast cell activation? Is it all the above? Is it mold toxins? We still don't fully understand why the NK cells are low. [But] we have had patients, with the transfer factors, be it Multi-Immune or some combination of them, in which the [NK cells] have come up. I've seen a couple of pretty dramatic ones in the last year or two. [I think] Researched Nutritionals even has a small study of NK cells going to normal with the Multi-Immune. [So] I still think the best thing to try is the transfer factor. Some of those combinations they have for NK cells."

Bob: "On the patients who go to zero mold, do you see … We talked about this before. Do you see the natural killer cells come back in everybody, or just in some?" Dr. Brewer: "I haven't tracked the natural killer cells that much in mold patients. I can't tell you."

Q: I've read that viruses can't be killed off.
a. So can you have viral die-off? Like in treating HHV-6 or EBV with an antiviral like valacyclovir. Or does such a treatment have a Herx-like reaction that merely mimics bacterial or fungal die-off symptoms?
b. Can you have a die-off type reaction on the PlasMyc Transfer Factor?

A: "The viral die-off … They talk about this in the literature, and I guess what they're saying is, that the active virus — the reproducing active virus — is actually dying off. But the dormant DNA is not. That's what stays in your system dormant, the virus DNA inside of a cell." Bob: "So you do get a die-off reaction?" Dr. Brewer: "Yes. We've seen it; I've seen it with transfer … I've probably seen it the least with transfer factor. But I've definitely seen it with valacyclovir, valganciclovir; I've seen it with the antivirals. And I'm not alone. Other doctors have, too. One of the docs out at … Stanford reported a lot of die-off in the patients he treated with valganciclovir."

Bob: "When I was looking back at 2016, when I was taking the valacyclovir, and I stopped it. And I didn't realize it at the time, but it was making me so much sicker because of die-off." Dr. Brewer: "Yes." Bob: "So after a bit, I did go back on it, and it did make me feel better." Dr. Brewer: "I think you've figured it out over the years. When you get die-off, adjust those doses. Come down on the doses. A lot of my people, if they feel too rough on say like a gram twice a day, they cut down to a half a gram once or twice a day. So that's the way you want to handle die-off is cut back on the dosing." Bob: "Yes, okay." Dr. Brewer: "It didn't sound like you had too much of it back in June when you were doing it. It sounded like you just maybe got a little bit better." Bob: "Sometimes it's just hard to figure out what's going on." Dr. Brewer: "No, I understand. I feel for you." We both laughed.

Bob: "I do feel much better since changing my diet, with the help of my friend. And that's why I think I can go back on the valacyclovir without a problem." Dr. Brewer: "I think you're right. When did you change the diet?" Bob: "Just a couple of days ago. Well, I changed it, we changed it a month ago. I took some stuff away that I thought was a good idea. Then we changed it again this weekend." Dr. Brewer: "But it's all been very recent?" Bob: "Yes. And it's helped with my liver pain." Dr. Brewer: "Cool.

Q: MCAS.

a. When I look at my immediate family, my parents and my brother never had major health issues before they reached their late 60s. And in my cousins' six member family, two had colon cancer in their 40s and 50s, but they both fully recovered and weren't sickly again until they got much older. So is it possible my MCAS is not genetic in nature?

b. It feels like my MCAS is under control for now. If it is, I would think it's because of the things I take for my liver. I try and eat organic as much a possible, and I've settled on some essential oils for my liver, all of which contain flavonoids — celery seed, turmeric, and yuzu (an oil from a Japanese citrus fruit). Is it possible my MCAS is under control, and by the methods mentioned?

A: Dr. Brewer: "So that kind of brings us to the MCAS. Usually we think dietary changes may have something to do with MCAS. Certainly people who have food allergies, or food intolerances, or gluten intolerances, or whatever …

"You've got to remember that there are billions, if not trillions, of mast cells in your GI tract; all the way from your mouth, all the way to the other end, there are mast cells everywhere in your GI tract. And so, whenever you eat something, it's going to come into contact with mast cells. And so we've had a number of mast cell patients that have had fairly dramatic changes with their diet. Unfortunately, it's not one size fits all. So it depends on what they're sensitive to. It will vary a lot from patient to patient. It sounds like your mast cell is doing pretty well.

"On the other hand, this dietary thing that you just told me about does sound like a mast cell-type issue. You've probably heard where people eat certain foods and they feel like they get inflamed. And that's somehow the immune cells — likely the mast cells in the gut — reacting to whatever the food is that is triggering it."

Bob: "Well, the stuff that I was getting rid of was probably stuff affecting my fatty liver." Dr. Brewer: "Yes. You know, fatty liver is highly associated with inflammation. That's basically what the fat does in the liver, it triggers inflammation.

"Your question about the genetic nature of mast cell activation, I mean that's another one that's not fully worked out. One of the things, and this may fit with your family, one of the things that's been shown with mast cell activation is, it can be sort of a dormant gene, if you will. It's kind of a dormant thing that just sits there for 30, 40, 50 years, and then it comes on at a later age. Because there's people who …

"I have people who never had allergies or anything for 45 or 50 years; and then, when they got some sort of a triggering event

— like a viral infection, or a car wreck, or whatever that triggered their CFS, fibromyalgia — now all of a sudden their skin breaks out; they have all kinds of allergies; etc. I've even seen that in some mold cases. They were never allergic to anything their whole life. [Then] once they got heavily exposed to mold, it seems to have triggered their mast cells. Now they're allergic to everything."

Bob: "So you're saying, like in my family, maybe the mast cells didn't activate until later in their lives?" Dr. Brewer: "Yes." Bob: "But with me, it activated because of the mold?" Dr. Brewer: "Yes. And we're saying, genetically, in medicine we call it genotype and phenotype. Genotype means that you've got the genetic genes there, but they may not be doing their thing. They may not be active. Phenotype means you then develop the symptoms and so forth."

Bob: "One other question. I guess this is a foolish question." We had some phone breakup here. "After I had that operation in the hospital, I came home and I was eating sandwiches. So I started eating chips with the sandwiches, and that's one of the things I cut out [of my diet recently]. My friend said, 'You've got to realize [the chips] are fried and can affect your fatty liver.' Is that true? I assume it's true." We got cut off again. Dr. Brewer: "So this was after your bladder surgery?" Bob: "Yes. So, since I am feeling better getting off those, maybe …" Dr. Brewer: "Yes." Bob: "So that would be like a fried food then?" Dr. Brewer: "Yes." Bob: "I don't know why I got back [to eating chips again, and so often]. Well, it was just simple. So it's a good thing I cut them out?" Dr. Brewer: "Agreed. Totally agree.

Q: A friend told me he self-published a book of his memoirs on https://www.amazon.com for $750. I think, at that price, my book on our visits may just come to fruition. Some questions:

a. Do you want your name on the book's cover in some capacity? (I will be using a pen name.)
b. Do you want to see a copy of the book when it's done and before I submit it to Amazon?
c. Is the doctor still okay with me doing this book? Does he think it would be worthwhile?

A: Dr. Brewer: "On your Amazon book, it's probably best not to have my name on the cover since I didn't participate in writing it." Bob: "That's what I figured." Dr. Brewer: "I would encourage you, if you can do it, I applaud you." Bob: "I still see all this stuff out there about, maybe it's thyroid, maybe it's this or that. I don't know. [Inaudible.] Like it helped my friend in California. He was in a nursing home. I gave him your information. He went to Dr. Nathan's old clinic in Sacramento. There's a doctor there that treated him with the antifungals. He's completely well; got his own apartment …"

Dr. Brewer: "Wow. Isn't that cool." Bob: "Yes, it's great. He used your information." Dr. Brewer: "That is great." Bob: "It would be the same information [my friend used to get healthy again] that would be in this book. I think there's a need for it. I don't know if anybody would read it, but …" Dr. Brewer: "Well, you know, put it out there and somebody will." Bob: "I would think so. There's enough people I would think that are desperate for this kind of help, like my friend was."

Q & A: Dr. Brewer: "So the last question is, am I retiring soon? No. I'm still not sure, but I'm going to work a few more years." Bob: "Okay. I just realized, you're starting to get up there." Dr. Brewer: "In six months, we'll have another appointment." Bob: "Okay. Sounds good." Dr. Brewer: "Assuming nothing happens with me, and I'm not anticipating it. And 'No,' you are not the first person to have asked." Bob: "Okay."

Dr. Brewer: "So I like the valacyclovir idea a lot. I like what you're doing with your diet. Keep playing with that; maybe let this friend help guide you on some of this stuff." Bob: "Yes, she's been pretty good."

Dr. Brewer: "Alright." Bob: "Alright. Thanks, Dr. Brewer." Dr. Brewer: "Oh. And also, if you don't feel better with the … Let's give the valacyclovir maybe about three months. But we should consider repeating the HHV-6 test maybe in three to six months if you're not feeling better."

<u>Phone Call on December 3, 2020:</u>

I got a phone call on this date from my friend Steve in California. Steve reported that, after 20 years, his natural killer cells had gone up from 1 to 9 — with 7 being the lowest number in the normal range. He was very excited about this. I told him that I thought it was possible he would see his NK cells go up even further down the road.

[In the *Natural Killer Cell, Functional* lab test by Quest Diagnostics, the normal range for the NK cells is 7 to 125.]

<u>Three Items in January 2021</u>:
Note: One definition of a tincture is that it is a concentrated herbal extract soaked in alcohol, with the alcohol content generally running from 25% to 60% of the total mixture. It is usually administered in drops. As I do with my homeopathic medicines, I add the drops of any tincture to a small amount of filtered water, and then I let it stand for 10 minutes before drinking it. I've read, and have been taught, that this is done to allow the alcohol to evaporate prior to dosing. (Although I sometimes wonder how much evaporation actually occurs.)

I've also read that you should avoid eating or drinking 10 to 15 minutes before and after taking your tincture (or homeopathic remedy).

I should mention that alcohol-free tinctures are sold as well. These often contain vegetable glycerin (a sugar-like substitute made from plant oils) and purified water. ~~

(1) I remembered that I used to take tinctures for medical conditions. This was one way to take a small dose of a herb, one

that didn't contain excipients and fillers as in a supplement. (I had even forgotten that I had tried the two Beyond Balance tinctures as recently as 2019).

So I started taking Holy Basil in a tincture to aid my kidneys, and bromelain in a tincture to aid my bladder. I am hopeful these tinctures, taken once a day, will calm any MCAS activity in those organs and help them to function better.

(2) Dr. Brewer had, in November 2020, talked about inflammation being associated with my kidney pain. Because I use so many essential oils, I don't know why it didn't dawn on me right away that there were plenty of oils that could help treat inflammation. So I made up a blend of three anti-inflammatory essential oils, lightly diluted in a carrier oil, which I now apply over my kidneys once every other day.

(3) Also around this time, in a phone call with my friend Steve, he told me the https://qnlabs.com website has supplements that contain no excipients. I went on the website and looked at a few supplements and their "other ingredients." Those other ingredients that I saw listed were things like *organic jasmine rice bran* and *vegetable cellulose capsules*. All the ingredients I saw looked harmless enough to me, so I may try some of their supplements one day. I also looked for quercetin and bioflavonoids, but I didn't see anything listed. Still, this may be a source of quality supplements for those with mast cell issues.

<u>FaceTime Visit #31 with Dr. Brewer on May 13, 2021:</u>

In my notes for the doctor [which was submitted five or six days ahead of time]:

<u>HHV-6/ EBV Activity Since My Last Visit November 17, 2020:</u>
a. November 18, 2020: I started back on the valacyclovir, alternating between one full tablet on one day and half a tablet the next day.
b. December 10, 2020: I began feeling pretty good.
c. February 28: after 102 days, I stopped the valacyclovir — much like I did in March 2017, when I had a lot of die-off. I began taking Researched Nutritionals Toxin-Pul, at one capsule every other day, to help with detox.
d. March 11: I started on one capsule every other day of the Multi-Immune Transfer Factor.
e. March 12: I went on half a capsule of the PlasMyc every other day, alternating with the Multi-Immune.
f. April 9: my HHV-6 test came back as still positive, at 11,600 cpy/mL, and I went back on half a tab of the valacyclovir daily. My EBV test appeared to still be elevated as well.

After a review of my file and my notes, the doctor asked me when we had done my last mold test, and I told him it was back in August 2020.   We then discussed my being on the valacyclovir, and the Multi-Immune and PlasMyc supplements.

Q. With the intranasal antifungal treatment, has the doctor stuck with the colloidal silver? Has that been as good a treatment as the doctor had hoped for back in May 2018?

A. "I'm not exclusively using colloidal silver, but I still use a lot of it. I had a really cool case this week. This is a lady I've followed for a long time. Kind of a weird story. She's been doing pretty well, up through about last September. So she called up in the fall, and of course last year Covid messed up everything. So she called up in the fall and said, 'I seem to be having all of these, this sinus infection; I've got all this problem in my sinuses, and congestion and pain and pressure. Then I'm so fatigued and wiped out, and I've got brain fog.' …

"She probably had five Covid tests, because everybody kept saying this must be Covid. But they were all negative. So we tried her on multiple different antibiotics and nothing worked. We tried her on amoxicillin, and a Z-Pac, and all these different antibiotics, and nothing worked. This carried on through about January or February.

"So then she calls up to my nurse, after the first of the year, and said, 'You know, I wonder if this could be mold?' Now she didn't have any reason to suspect mold. She had it in her house years ago. She got heavily, heavily exposed [in a house] she had down near Gardner, Kansas. She got terribly exposed. But then she ultimately sold that house. Now it turns out we think she was exposed recently, but at the time she called she wasn't aware of anything. But she said, 'You know, maybe I ought to try that nasal spray again.' And I can't remember if we did a urine test on her or not.

"Anyway, she started on the colloidal silver nasal spray, and she just told me this week it was like a miracle. … She had phenomenal results with it. I mean, she said, 'I'm back to my old self again.' And it occurred quickly. She said, after she started on the nasal spray, she felt better within three days. So, you know, that's not going to apply to everybody. So anyway, it was a fascinating story.

"But I do have some people who haven't been great responders to the colloidal silver. I still use some nasal nystatin, some of those. I would say, most often I've used colloidal silver, but I still use some of the others as well. Some of them that you've taken before."

Bob: "At one point, you hoped that maybe the colloidal silver would get rid of the mold all together. Did you ever find that to be true?" Dr. Brewer: " I don't think so. I think it grows back." Bob: "Just like with the nystatin?" Dr. Brewer: "Yes. And it's those darn spores. Because, you know, mold formed spores, they are heat resistant, cold resistant, drying resistant … Spores can live in nature for probably a 1,000 years. They're hard to kill.

Dr. Brewer: "Now let's talk about the EBV and HHV-6. Sir, we still have a problem with you. You still got HHV-6 floating around." Bob: "Yes." Dr. Brewer: "The numbers not as high, but it's still there.

After some talk about the Covid vaccines and the herpes viruses, we got back to the HHV-6.

Dr. Brewer: "So I have a lady that's about your age, and she's a Lyme and a mold case. And she has found that she does the best if she stays on a low dose antibiotic like amoxicillin for Lyme. And we've given her several rounds of mold treatment, and that's gone pretty well.

"So she had been doing really good for probably a year and a half, two years. So last September, out of the blue, for no good reason that we can come up with, she crashed. Now she may have had some mold exposure, but it was brief. Again, this was in September. So she said, 'Do you think it's my Lyme?' And I said, 'I don't think so. You're on the same antibiotic as before; we haven't changed anything.' So we weren't coming up with much.

"So she calls in one day and talks with my nurse, and said, 'Dr. Brewer had checked me for EBV and HHV-6 back about 2016, '17, somewhere in there, and I was very high in HHV-6. Could we recheck those?' So I reordered them. And actually, her HHV-6 — now this is not the PCR test that you had done, this is the antibody levels — and so her HHV-6 was actually lower that it was three or four years ago.

"But she said, 'You know, Dr. Brewer talked about trying me on valganciclovir back then, and we ran it through my insurance'

— she's about your age, so it's Medicare Part D — and we ran it through her insurance, and it wouldn't cover it. I mean, it was going to be like over a $1,000 out-of-pocket." Bob: "Whoa!" Dr. Brewer: "That's why I've never even thought about it with you, because insurance usually doesn't cover it, and it's big time out-of-pocket. So she said, 'I'm going to look into it again.'

"So she calls back, in about a week, and she says, 'I've found a Good Rx coupon where I can get it for like, I think, under $200.' Okay? So she says, 'So can Dr. Brewer send me a prescription.' Now this was December, maybe January. Right around the first of the year. So she calls back two weeks later and all of her symptoms are gone." Bob: "Wow." Dr. Brewer: "Oh, this is even better. One pill once a day." Bob: "Wow." Dr. Brewer: "So she's been fine. So we treated her for three months. Stopped it about April 1. And she just called back last week, and her symptoms have come back again, and she wants me to prescribe it again. Which I did. So the interesting part is, for most people historically, particularly with Medicare Part D, the valganciclovir has been unaffordable."

Bob: "When I changed my drug plan at the end of the year, I made sure that both of those were covered, both of those drugs, so …" Dr. Brewer: "Valganciclovir's covered?" Bob: "Yes. But my co-pay is like $150 a month." Dr. Brewer: "Can you afford that?" Bob: "Yes. If I have to." Dr. Brewer: "Okay. Do you want to try it?" Bob: "I'd rather stay on the valacyclovir right now, because I did so well with it in 2017." I then reminded the doctor I had restarted the valacyclovir April 9. Dr. Brewer: "So you've been on it about a month."

Bob: "Yes, but I'm taking a small dose. I was thinking I might try to up either the immune booster — of course, I don't know if I'm going to continue to feel better, but I'm feeling a lot better the last two days — so I was thinking about maybe boosting one of the transfer factors. And then, if I do okay, maybe boosting the valacyclovir." Dr. Brewer: "Yes, I'm fine with that plan." Bob: "Then if I don't get better, contact you and get a prescription for the valganciclovir."

Dr. Brewer: "I agree. I like your plan. … So you're going to stick with the valacyclovir; play around a little bit with the immune factors, and then you'll let me know if you want the valganciclovir. Correct?"

Bob: "Yes. I remember there were some, didn't you say there were some problems with that? You had to have your blood monitored, or something, with the valganciclovir?" Dr. Brewer: "Yes, but just like once a month." Bob: "That's a lot. You have to have blood work once a month?" Dr. Brewer: "Yes, for the first month or two. Yes." Bob: "Okay." Dr. Brewer: "Don't you have, do you have a service down in Lawrence where they'll come and draw it at your house?" Bob: "No. They used to, before the pandemic."

Dr. Brewer: "Some of them are doing it again. Let me say, here in Kansas City there's a service that will do it. Now I think this is all going to go away anyway because of the vaccines,

[with] so many people [having] been vaccinated and so forth. But the lady would actually come and do it in the driveway, or the garage." Bob: "I had Visiting Physicians, and they would come and draw blood themselves, but they went out of business in Kansas City at the end of the year. There's another doctor in Kansas City that is starting up a similar thing, but they don't have any patients in Lawrence yet. So I told them, 'You get more patients, I'll sign up.'"

Dr. Brewer: "Don't worry about it. I mean, we can maybe even wait six weeks. I'm not going to say you can take it without getting blood work drawn, but it's not real rigid on how frequently we have to get it."

Bob: "How many tablets would you prescribe, and how many …" Dr. Brewer: "The lady — now you know, you're bigger than she is, just in body weight and so forth, and you're a male instead of a female — but the lady that we did it with, she just took one pill a day. Which of course is going to cut back on the cost. And I would say, start there. One pill a day."

Bob: "Okay. I hope my feeling better lasts, so I can go ahead and get back …" Dr. Brewer: "Me, too. I hope this two days is going to lead to a whole lot of good days."

FaceTime Visit #32 with Dr. Brewer on November 9, 2021:

<u>(a) Another View on Mold and Toxic Mold:</u>

I finally got around to reading *Through the Shadowlands* by the science writer Julie Rehmeyer. In the book, she detailed her own experience with CFS and toxic mold. She doesn't have the toxic mold colonization problem in her nasal passages, but instead she is very reactive to any mold and mold toxin exposure. I asked Dr. Brewer about this.

Q. Does the doctor know, or have an idea, why CFS patients who the doctor treats for toxic mold are like/unlike those CFS patients who do well with mold-avoidance (those who get very ill, very quickly when they're exposed to the least bit of mold)?

A. "I think some people are just exquisitely sensitive to mold, and probably not just the toxins. Some of them, it's the toxins; some of them, it's the actual mold itself; and some of them, it's both. Because the toxins are chemical products that are made by the mold, and not all mold makes toxins."

Bob: "They can be very sensitive to the mold, but they don't get that mold in the nasal passages, that colonization?"

Dr. Brewer: "Correct. Basically, I think some people … We kind of use the word allergic, they're allergic to it. Now, it may not be classic allergy where they break out in hives, or have asthma, or that sort of thing. Some of my patients who are mast cell patients, who have a lot of allergies, they will openly say their number one problem is mold."

Note: There is a Mold Avoiders website at: https:// moldavoiders.com.

<u>(b) The return of the HHV-6:</u>
I discussed with Dr. Brewer how I had been feeling knocked out all summer, and by the end of September I had also started feeling sickly again as well. Then I told the doctor I wanted to try the drug valganciclovir, for active HHV-6 infection, which we had previously discussed. Dr. Brewer said I had tested positive for HHV-6 two or three times in the past, which obviously wasn't normal. Then he said, "I'm going to order the test for the HHV-6. And I'll go ahead and send a prescription to your pharmacy for valganciclovir."

Bob: "And you said before that, after four weeks on the valganciclovir, I would need to do a blood test?" Dr. Brewer: "Yes." He said I should contact his nurse in a month and ask her to order the test for me to be done at my local lab.

<u>Following My Visit with the Doctor:</u>
I took my HHV-6 test on November 11, 2021, and the results came back two months later. I had 19,300 copies/ml, and as Dr. Brewer had previously said, "It should be less than 1,000."

I also received the prescription for the valganciclovir on November 11, 2021. The dosage was 450 mg to be taken once a day; and with my drug plan coverage, it cost me $28 for a two month's supply. I started the prescription the same day I received it, and I had stayed on it until February 20, 2022 — a period of 106 days. I had stopped the valganciclovir when I had become much more ill, which I suspected was from viral die-off because it resembled my experience back in 2017 from being on the valacyclovir.

After another office visit on May 3, 2022, Dr. Brewer ordered a new HHV-6 test for me. I received the results in the first week of July, and it showed I now had 4,020 copies/ml. While that was still in the infection range, I felt comfortable that I didn't need to go back on the valganciclovir.

<u>Chapter Nine: My Recovery</u>

<u>The Mold Returns, July 2022:</u>

Because I didn't seem to be doing any better after the HHV-6 treatment, and with Dr. Brewer on board, I sent in a new toxic mold test, and I got those results back July 11, 2022. In that test, all my mold numbers were up substantially.

Since my mold numbers had mostly been drifting downward since 2016, I theorized that my mold numbers were back up again because the original antifungal treatment had killed the mold down substantially but not completely; and then the mold just took the last few years to grow back in strength. Of course, I planned to ask Dr. Brewer if my theory was correct the next time I saw him.

In any event, when my test results came in, Dr. Brewer suggested I go back on the nasal antifungal medication, and I agreed. This time, I was going to try the colloidal silver nasal antifungal; and this time, I planned that, after my mold numbers came back down again, I would stay on a maintenance dose of the nasal antifungal after that.

So this illustrates a very important point. Dr. Brewer has said many times before, because it is almost impossible to kill off all the toxic mold in the nasal passages, that after their initial mold treatment, most of his patients have had to go on a maintenance dose of the nasal antifungals for the rest of their lives. This was necessary in order to keep the patient's mold toxin activity at bay.

Mold Test in December 2023:

After over a year on my new mycotoxin therapy, I got my latest RealTime Labs mycotoxin test back. Virtually all my my mold toxins were no longer present. Dr. Brewer wrote and told me I could now go on a maintenance dose of the colloidal silver, which he said was one dose twice a week.

Update in September 2024:

At this time, I found that my CFS was finally in remission. This allowed me to stop taking all my supplements, oils, tinctures, and homeopathic medicines that got me through each day with my CFS, except those for my heart and liver. (By mid-November, I was able to stop all those medicines for my heart and liver as well).

When looking back on my symptoms of mid-2011, many of them were now gone. My mold toxin levels were low, and my MCAS seemed under control. Unfortunately, being 79 years old, I now had health issues I was dealing with other than my CFS.

Here is where I stood then, as of this update:

Changes in my old symptoms: (a) fatigue with my other health issues is a feeling of being very tired, but it is not the bone-crushing fatigue of CFS as I once described it to Dr. Brewer, and (b) shortness of breath, sleep disturbances, poor balance, and muscle weakness are from other health issues.

Symptoms I no longer have: (a) post-exertional malaise, (b) brain fog, and (c) dizziness, headaches, digestive issues, and muscle spasms. As per the brain fog, my short term memory is good once again, as is my cognitive function.

Remaining issues I have: (a) liver damage, (b) aerobic exercise still makes me feel much worse, but anaerobic exercise is still okay, and (c) multiple chemical sensitivity, though it's not as bad as it was before.

Issues that should correct over time: (a) my immune system should go back to normal, as it did with my friend Steve, and (b) I would expect my diastolic heart dysfunction to also correct.

<u>Telehealth Visit #36 with Dr. Brewer on December 11, 2024:</u>

As the visit began, I told Dr. Brewer that my CFS was finally in remission. And then I added: "THANK YOU!"

<u>My Diastolic Heart Dysfunction:</u>

Bob: "So I'm wondering, now that the mold is down, could my diastolic heart failure resolve, because wasn't that the mitochondria being attacked by the mold in the heart kind of making your heart weak and not functioning properly?"

Dr. Brewer: "We don't know. … I wouldn't think so, but your reasoning is not bad. We know that mold can attack the mitochondria, and the mitochondria [are probably not] functioning normally in the diastolic heart. Now the question is, does mold have anything to do with the cause of diastolic heart failure? I think it's doubtful, but it's possible. Are they going to do another echo at some point?"

Bob: "I assume so. … I would mention this. You know, I was taking massive amounts of ubiquinol for my heart, which you put me on 12 years ago. Well, I'm not taking ubiquinol anymore, and my chest pain hasn't come back. That's why I was asking about maybe the heart could correct, the diastolic problem." Dr. Brewer: "Right. Interesting. They'll be able to tell when they do an echo down the line."

<u>A Delayed Reaction:</u>

At one point in my visit, I said to Dr. Brewer: "I don't why there was such a delayed reaction from my mold numbers being low in December [2023] to my not fully feeling [that my CFS was in remission] until September [2024]."

Dr. Brewer: "I've seen it before, where there's kind of a slower trickle of feeling better, and then it finally catches up and the patient feels better. I've seen that before."

<u>Chapter Ten: OTC Nasal Sprays</u>

In April of 2025, it came to my attention that people who wanted to get tested for toxic mold, and treated for the toxic mold if they had it, were hard pressed to find a treating physician. Mostly because these types of doctors are rare; but more so because the few medical doctors that are out there that treat toxic mold don't take insurance, and they also charge a lot of money for their medical care.

As for the RealTime Labs test, E8400 MYCO16 Panel, people can order that for themselves, if they are willing to pay the full price for the test.

As for the colloidal silver that had helped me, the main thing I found out was that the "Elemental Silver" (or silver in its pure form), the drug in my last nasal antifungal prescription, had a $+1$ charge, which is what makes it effective in fighting microbial growths. However, I read that when the silver is placed in some colloidal solutions, the charge can turn neutral, and thus it can lose its therapeutic value.

I next looked for over-the-counter (OTC) antifungal nasal sprays that people might be able to purchase and use on their own. What I found is below, including the information of my colloidal silver nasal spray from PD Labs.

The colloidal silver that was prescribed for me was from PD Labs; and it is called "ACS Nasal Spray," and it contains 30 ppm of "Elemental Silver" in "Ultra Pure deionized water." To this, you as the patient add a biofilm buster that comes included separately with the prescription.

Then there is the OTC "Biofilm Clear Nasal Spray." The website for this product, at https://www.biofilmclear.com/, says it contains colloidal silver, along with three biofilm busters: EDTA, Xylitol, and Grapefruit Extract. The website also says that it is "Recommended for Shoemaker Protocol." In a chat on the Internet, a person who identified themselves as the founder of the company told me that their product contained 30 ppm of colloidal silver. That they use "pharma grade nano colloidal silver in our spray from a vendor who is FDA certified. Our product is manufactured for us in a FDA certified facility too, who also tests all ingredients in the formula for purity and contaminants."

In later emails with the company, I was told this product contains both Ionic silver (the positively charged silver) and Nano-silver, both suspended in water, and both of which are necessary to ensure potency and shelf life. In addition, I was told that this "product uses distilled water, which contains extremely low levels of ions and impurities, providing a clean, stable base that won't interfere with the silver particles." Finally, I was told that each batch of BioFilm Clear is tested for microbiological purity before release and meets USP standards to ensure safety and consistency.

Lastly, there is the "Argentyn 23," and it contains 23 ppm of colloidal silver. The website at https://argentyn23.com/ says this is a "Bio-Active Silver Hydrosol" that has only two ingredients: 99.999% pure silver, and water that meets USP-NF standards for pharmaceutical-grade purified water." That the product has a "Positive Charge - Greater than 98% bio-active silver ions and nanoclusters."

I have seen the usage of the Argentyn 23 talked about by Dr. Neil Nathan on a YouTube video. However, it does not appear to contain a biofilm buster. I found an OTC biofilm buster called "Xlear Nasal Spray," and it's available on amazon.com. It contains purified water, USP sodium chloride, and the biofilm busters Xylitol and Grapefruit Seed Extract.

Note 1: Bio-Active Silver Hydrosol is a mixture of silver ions and silver nanoclusters (the smallest particles achievable).

Note 2: According to the USP-NF website at https://www.uspnf.com/, "The USP–NF is a combination of two compendia, the United States Pharmacopeia (USP) and the National Formulary (NF). It contains standards for medicines, dosage forms, drug substances, excipients, biologics, compounded preparations, medical devices, dietary supplements, and other therapeutics. USP is an independent, scientific nonprofit organization focused on building trust in the supply of safe, quality medicines."

Note 3: As a FYI. In July of 2025, in an email to BioFilm Clear users, the company announced a new partnership between it and MoldCo, a Telehealth provider focused on mold-related lab testing and treatment options for mold-related conditions. The email said MoldCo had two mold tests available.

Apparently sold at cost, "MoldCo's Starter Mold Panel tests 3 key biomarkers (MSH, MMP-9, and TGF-β1) for just \$99. This panel offers a valuable starting point for identifying possible biotoxin exposure and tracking your treatment response." Then, with a discount code offering \$150 off, "MoldCo also offers a Complete Panel testing 16 biomarkers."

The email said "these lab tests can offer helpful guidance and a clear baseline to track your progress." ~~

If the information I have received is honest, and as a layman with no medical training, it looks like to me the two OTC colloidal silver nasal sprays mentioned could be effective in killing off toxic mold when it is present in the nasal passages of CFS patients. But anyone interested in this OTC nasal spray therapy should first do their own research in this area, and then consult on this with any medical professionals they currently work with or can gain access to.

For anyone on Dr. Brewer's treatment protocol for toxic mold, whether using prescription antifungals or OTC colloidal silver, there is a subreddit where they can go to discuss their treatment and talk with others who have similar interests. The subreddit is: r/cfsFibroTreatment.

<u>Chapter Eleven: Sign Off</u>

Disclaimer: As the author of this writing, I want to state that I am not a medical doctor, nor have I ever been employed in the medical field in any capacity.

Still, I have tried to describe important medical information on the disease of CFS as told to me by my infectious disease doctor. It is my hope that this book and its information, in some way, can help others who suffer from this illness.

I am also not a professional writer. I should add that, as to the content of this book, I considered various options for editing it differently. But in the end, I decided I had no idea what the situation might be for various possible readers. So I just told my experience in as straightforward a manner as I could.

Should you wish to contact me, you can find me posting on the subreddit r/cfsFibroTreatment.

Signed,
Robert Roy